MEDICAL TERMINOLOGY CONCEPTS

A Review Guide

Lisa L. Campbell, Ph.D.

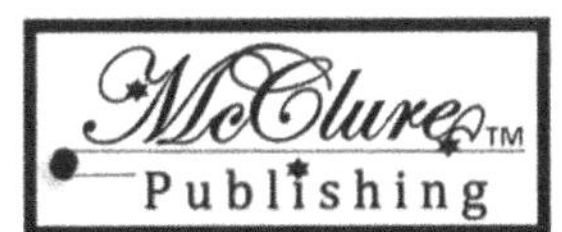

McClure Publishing, Inc.
www.McClurePublishing.com

ISBN-13: 979-8-9853967-6-8

To order additional copies, please contact:

McClure Publishing, Inc.
www.mcclurepublishing.com
800.659.4908

Lisa L. Campbell, Ph.D.
Physician Practice Resources, Inc.
www.drlisalcampbell.org
855.737.5472

Medical Terminology Concepts:
A Review Guide

Dr. Lisa L. Campbell, PhD
RHIA, CDIP, CCS, CCS-P,
CPC, COC, CPB, CRC, CPMA, CPC-I

Dr. Campbell is a multi-faceted health care professional with 30 years of experience. Having a passion for working with physician practices, Dr. Campbell enjoys helping providers improve their operational effectiveness with a focus on documentation integrity.

She holds professional memberships with the American Health Information Management Association (AHIMA), American Academy of Professional Coders (AAPC) and Association of Clinical Documentation Improvement Specialists (ACDIS).

She holds a Masters in Health Administration (MHA), Masters in Project Management (MPM) and Doctor of Philosophy (PhD) degree in Health Care Administration. Additionally, she holds the following nationally recognized credentials:

- Registered Health Information Administrator (RHIA)
- Certified Documentation Improvement Practitioner (CDIP)
- Certified Coding Specialist (CCS)
- Certified Coding Specialist-Physician Based (CCS-P)
- Certified Professional Coder (CPC)
- Certified Outpatient Coder (COC)
- Certified Professional Biller (CPB)
- Certified Risk Coder (CRC)
- Certified Professional Medical Auditor (CPMA)
- Certified Professional Coder-Instructor (CPC-I)

Lastly, Dr. Campbell has been an educator since 1997 on-campus and online, for several Colleges and Universities across the United States.

Table of Contents

Chapter 1-Prefixes

A prefix is a term added before a medical term and is used to alter its meaning and form a new word. Using the list of terms below, create flash cards to learn the meaning of each prefix, prior to completing the assessment that follows.

a-
ab-
ad-
an-
ana-
ante-
anti-
auto-
bi-
brady-
cata-
con-
contra-
de-
dia-
ec-
ecto-
endo-
epi-
eu-
ex-
exo-
hemi-
hyper-
hypo-

in-
infra-
inter-
macro-
mal-
meta-
neo-
pan-
per-
peri-
poly-
post-
pre-
pros-
pseudo-
re-
retro-
sub-
sym-
syn-
tachy-
trans-
ultra-
uni-

Multiple Choice

Circle the most appropriate response.

_____ 1. **The prefix that means no; not; without**
A) a-, an-
B) endo-
C) intra -
D) eu-

_____ 2. **The prefix that means on, upon, over is**
A) intra-
B) pro-
C) epi-
D) sub-

_____ 3. **The prefix that means through, complete is**
A) dia-
B) hyper-
C) dys-
D) pro-

_____ 4. **The prefix exo- is defined as**
A) out
B) away from
C) in
D) a and b

_____ 5. **The prefix that means in; within**
A) exo-
B) ex-
C) endo-
D) epi-

_____ 6. **The prefix that means out is**
A) ex-
B) epi-
C) endo-
D) a and b

_____ 7. **The prefix that means excessive**
A) hypo-
B) hyper-
C) sub-
D) trans-

_____ 8. **The prefix that means deficient; below; under**
A) trans-
B) hyper-
C) hypo-
D) pro-

_____ 9. **The prefix that means surrounding is**
A) endo-
B) pro-
C) peri-
D) hypo-

_____ 10. **The prefix that means before; forward**
A) sub-
B) pros-
C) retro-
D) re

_____ 11. **The prefix re- means**
A) back
B) again
C) backward
D) all of the above

_____ 12. **The prefix retro- means**
A) back
B) backward
C) behind
D) all of the above

_____ 13. **The prefix that means below,under is**
A) sub-
B) trans-
C) re-
D) peri-

____ **14. The prefix that means through, across**
A) epi-
B) endo-
C) trans-
D) path-

____ **15. The prefix that means self is**
A) bi-
B) auto-
C) hetero-
D) none of the above

____ **16. The prefix that means two**
A) bio-
B) bi-
C) lateral-
D) tri-

____ **17. The prefix ec-, ecto- means**
A) in, inside
B) out, outside
C) in, out
D) all of the above

____ **18. The prefix that means new**
A) micro-
B) nulli-
C) micro-
D) neo-

____ **19. The prefix that means uni-**
A) one
B) two
C) three
D) five

____ **20. The prefix that means up, apart is**
A) ab-
B) ad-
C) ante-
D) ana-

____ **21. The prefix that means toward is**
- A) an-
- B) ad-
- C) ab-
- D) ana-

____ **22. The prefix poly- is defined as**
- A) many, much
- B) without
- C) through
- D) few

____ **23. The prefix that means away from is**
- A) a-
- B) an-
- C) ab-
- D) ad-

____ **24. The prefix that means against, opposite is**
- A) con-
- B) contra-
- C) cata-
- D) brady-

____ **25. The prefix that means against is**
- A) ante-
- B) anti-
- C) auto-
- D) cata-

____ **26. The prefix that means large**
- A) macro-
- B) mal-
- C) hemi-
- D) meta-

____ **27. The prefix hemi- is defined as**
- A) four
- B) half
- C) before
- D) two

____ 28. **The prefix that means bad is**
A) mal-
B) macro-
C) in-
D) meta-

____ 29. **The prefix that means with, together**
A) cata-
B) con-
C) contra-
D) brady-

____ 30. **The prefix that means beyond, excess**
A) ultra-
B) uni-
C) trans-
D) supra-

____ 31. **The prefix that means through**
A) per-
B) peri-
C) transit-
D) poly-

____ 32. **The prefix de- means**
A) down
B) up
C) lack of
D) a and c

____ 33. **The prefix that means near; beside**
A) neo-
B) para-
C) per-
D) meta-

____ 34. **The prefix that means before, in front of**
A) pre-
B) post-
C) meta-
D) supra-

____ **35. The prefix infra- means**
    A) into
    B) not
    C) between
    D) beneath

____ **36. The prefix that means false**
    A) pseudo-
    B) re-
    C) retro-
    D) sub

____ **37. The prefix that means slow**
    A) bi-
    B) brady-
    C) con-
    D) contra-

____ **38. The suffix -blast means**
    A) to blow up
    B) embryonic
    C) immature
    D) b and c only

____ **39. The prefix inter- means**
    A) holding
    B) between
    C) within
    D) connecting

____ **40. The prefix that means all**
    A) peri-
    B) pan-
    C) per-
    D) para-

____ **41. The prefix that means after, beyond, change, is**
    A) hyper-
    B) neo-
    C) hypo-
    D) meta-

____ 42. The prefix that means down
A) cata-
B) contra-
C) con-
D) brady-

____ 43. The prefix for together, with is
A) syn-
B) sym-
C) growth-
D) either a or b

____ 44. The prefix that means good, normal
A) normo-
B) eu-
C) ex-
D) brady-

____ 45. The prefix that means fast, rapid is
A) brady-
B) tachy-
C) hyper-
D) meta-

____ 46. The prefix that means into
A) endo-
B) peri-
C) in-
D) epi-

____ 47. The prefix that means after, behind
A) post-
B) peri-
C) para-
D) pan-

____ 48. The prefix ante- means
A) against
B) after
C) before
D) without

Chapter 2-Combining Forms

A word root coupled with a combining vowel, which may be separated in writing by a vertical slash is a combining from. Using the list of terms below, create flash cards to learn the meaning of each combining form, prior to completing the assessment that follows.

Aden/o
Arthr/o
Bi/o
Carcin/o
Cardi/o
Cephal/o
Cerebr/o
Cis/o
Crin/o
Cyst/o
Cyt/o
Derm/o
Dermat/o
Electr/o
Encephal/o
Enter/o
Erthyr/o
Gastr/o
Glyc/o
Gnos/o
Gynec/o

Hem/o
Hemat/o
Hepat/o
Iatr/o
Leuk/o
Log/o
Neur/o
Onc/o
Ophthalm/o
Oste/o
Path/o
Ped/o
Psych/o
Radi/o
Ren/o
Rhin/o
Sarc/o
Sect/o
Thromb/o
Ur/o

Multiple Choice

Circle the most appropriate response.

_____ 1. **The combining form hem/o, hemat/o means**
A) hemoglobin
B) hematocrit
C) blood
D) plasma

_____ 2. **The combining form ped/o means**
A) foot
B) child
C) pedicle
D) a and b

_____ 3. **The combining form aden/o means**
A) wrinkles
B) life
C) gland
D) scaly

_____ 4. **The combining form that means mind is**
A) men/o
B) ped/o
C) psych/o
D) all of the above

_____ 5. **The combining form ophthalm/o means**
A) lens
B) vision
C) eyelid
D) eye

_____ 6. **The combining form cis/o means to**
A) view
B) secrete
C) excise
D) cut

___ 7. The combining form that means red is
A) erthyr/o
B) xanth/o
C) leuk/o
D) melan/o

___ 8. The combining form that means bone is
A) my/o
B) arthr/o
C) synovi/o
D) oste/o

___ 9. The combining form for liver is
A) hepat/o
B) lingu/o
C) palat/o
D) uvul/o

___ 10. The combining form that means joint is
A) aponeur/o
B) arthr/o
C) burs/o
D) tendin/o

___ 11. The combining form thromb/o is defined as
A) sound
B) heat
C) electricity
D) clot

___ 12. The combining form cyst/o means
A) cell
B) urinary bladder
C) to secrete
D) female

___ 13. The combining form that means nerve is
A) hepat/o
B) neur/o
C) gastr/o
D) none of the above

____ **14. The combining form bi/o means**
A) two
B) life
C) death
D) three

____ **15. The combining form cardi/o means**
A) lung
B) liver
C) cards
D) heart

____ **16. The combining form that means kidney is**
A) nephr/o
B) vasic/o
C) ren/o
D) a and c

____ **17. The combining form iatr/o is defined as**
A) treatment
B) specialty
C) condition
D) a or b

____ **18. The combining form log/o means**
A) to study
B) one who studies
C) a specialist
D) knowledge

____ **19. A combining form is made up of a**
A) word root and combining vowel
B) prefix and combining vowel
C) combining vowel and suffix
D) prefix and word root

____ **20. The combining form cerebr/o means**
A) cerebrum
B) cerebellum
C) skull
D) a and b

____ 21. The combining form ur/o means
A) urine
B) urinary tract
C) water
D) a and b

____ 22. The combining form that means skin is
A) derm/o
B) dermatitis
C) dermat/o
D) a and c

____ 23. The combining form that means white is
A) erythr/o
B) cyan/o
C) xanth/o
D) leuk/o

____ 24. The combining form that means cell is
A) cyt/o
B) eti/o
C) hist/o
D) path/o

____ 25. The combining form crin/o means
A) endocrine gland
B) exocrine gland
C) secrete; separate
D) adrenal glad

____ 26. The combining form that means sugar is
A) hidr/o
B) hydr/o
C) glyc/o
D) a and c

____ 27. The combining form that means woman is
A) andr/o
B) uter/o
C) gynec/o
D) a and c

____ 28. The combining form carcin/o means
A) calcium
B) cancer
C) tumor
D) none of the above

____ 29. The combining form that means disease is
A) melan/o
B) path/o
C) carcin/o
D) eti/o

____ 30. The combining form that means brain is
A) cephal/o
B) encephal/o
C) psych/o
D) a and c

____ 31. The combining form onc/o means
A) eye
B) bone
C) tumor
D) cancer

____ 32. The combining form sect/o means
A) To make an artifical opening
B) To cut away
C) To cut
D) To make an incision

____ 33. The combining form rhin/o means
A) nose
B) sinus
C) septum
D) air

____ 34. The combining form that means head is
A) encephal/o
B) cephal/o
C) enter/o
D) cerebr/o

____ 35. The combining form that means stomach is
   A) somat/o
   B) stomat/o
   C) hepat/o
   D) gastr/o

____ 36. The combining form sarc/o means
   A) tumor
   B) cell
   C) flesh
   D) cancer

____ 37. The combining form electr/o means
   A) a record
   B) ECG
   C) electricity
   D) to record

____ 38. The combining form for intestines is
   A) col/o
   B) or/o
   C) ile/o
   D) enter/o

____ 39. The combining form that means knowledge is
   A) gastr/o
   B) glyc/o
   C) gnos/o
   D) gynec/o

____ 40. The combining form radi/o means
   A) radio
   B) radical
   C) x-rays
   D) all of the above

Chapter 3-Suffixes

A suffix is a term added to the end a medical term and is used to alter its meaning and form a new word. Using the list of terms below, create flash cards to learn the meaning of each prefix, prior to completing the assessment that follows.

-ac	-lysis
-al	-malacia
-algia	-megaly
-blast	-mission
-cele	-oid
-centesis	-ole
-coccus	-oma
-crine	-opsy
-cyesis	-osis
-cyte	-ostomy
-drome	-ous
-dynia	-partum
-ectomy	-pathy
-emia	-penia
-er	-phobia
-gen	-physis
-genesis	-plasia
-genic	-plasty
-globin	-pnea
-gram	-ptosis
-graphy	-rrhea
-ia	-sclerosis
-ic	-scope
-ical	-scopy
-ist	-stasis
-itis	-supra
-ium	-tomy
-lapse	-trophy
-logy	-um

Multiple Choice

Circle the most appropriate response.

____ 1. **The suffix -genic means**
A) pertaining to
B) genetics
C) produced by or in
D) a and c

____ 2. **The suffix that means pain is**
A) -cele
B) -pexy
C) -spasm
D) -algia

____ 3. **The suffix that means pertaining to is**
A) -ic, -ical
B) -ac, -al
C) -intra
D) a and b

____ 4. **The suffix that means viewing is**
A) -ia
B) -opsy
C) -plasty
D) b and c

____ 5. **The suffix -ectomy is defined as**
A) surgical repair
B) instrument used to cut
C) excision or surgical removal
D) a and c

____ 6. **The suffix -ist means**
A) pertaining
B) condition
C) specialist
D) study of

_____ **7. The suffix that means process is**
A) -ic
B) -logy
C) -ion
D) -ical

_____ **8. The suffix -cyte means**
A) excision
B) cell
C) blood condition
D) pain

_____ **9. The suffix that means blood condition is**
A) -ectomy
B) -oma
C) -emia
D) none of the above

_____ **10. The sufix -gram means**
A) process of recording
B) record
C) a and b
D) none of the above

_____ **11. The suffix that means inflammation is**
A) -ion
B) -ist
C) -itis
D) -logy

_____ **12. The suffix -logy means**
A) specialist
B) the study of
C) pertaining
D) biology

_____ **13. The suffix that means tumor is**
A) -opsy
B) -oma
C) -cyte
D) -al

____ **14. The suffix that means disease**
A) -ology
B) -pathy
C) -tomy
D) -ion

____ **15. The suffix that means condition is**
A) -itis
B) -osis
C) -pathy
D) -emia

____ **16. The suffix that means the process of viewing**
A) -scopy
B) -scope
C) -gram
D) -graphy

____ **17. The suffix that means the process of cutting**
A) -ostomy
B) -tomy
C) -ology
D) -scopy

____ **18. The suffix -scope means**
A) to remove
B) to record
C) instrument used to view
D) all of the above

____ **19. The suffix -globin means**
A) sugar
B) fat
C) protein
D) all of the above

____ **20. The suffix -malacia is defined as**
A) viewing
B) softening
C) eating
D) swallowing

____ 21. The suffix that means hernia
A) -cyte
B) -cele
C) -centesis
D) -coccus

____ 22. The suffix that means control, stop, place is
A) -osis
B) -plasm
C) -genesis
D) -stasis

____ 23. The suffix that means surgical puncture to aspirate fluid is
A) -capnia
B) -centesis
C) -tomy
D) either b or c

____ 24. The suffix that means fear
A) -phobia
B) -acro
C) -agora
D) none of the above

____ 25. The suffix that means surgical repair is
A) -angio
B) -plasty
C) -tomy
D) all of the above

____ 26. The suffix -um, ium mean
A) structure
B) tissue
C) thing
D) all of the above

____ 27. The suffix that means one who is
A) -ology
B) -er
C) -ia
D) -tic

____ **28. The suffix -plasia is defined as**
A) formation, development, growth
B) causing
C) eating
D) abnormal condition

____ **29. The suffix that means hardening is**
A) -malacia
B) -sclerosis
C) -penia
D) -crit

____ **30. The suffix that means producing; forming is**
A) -genesis
B) -ous
C) -gen
D) a and c

____ **31. The suffix -ptosis means**
A) drooping
B) sagging
C) proplase
D) all of the above

____ **32. The suffix that means pertaining to is**
A) -some
B) -ous
C) a and b
D) none of the above

____ **33. The suffix that means the process of recording**
A) -gram
B) -graph
C) -graphy
D) -all of the above

____ **34. The suffix that means berry shaped is**
A) -ia
B) -phagia
C) -coccus
D) -malacia

____ **35. The suffix that means deficiency is**
A) -algia
B) -penia
C) -sclerosis
D) -apharesis

____ **36. The suffix that means the process of viewing**
A) -scopy
B) -scope
C) -gram
D) -graphy

____ **37. The suffix that means nourishment, development is**
A) -esis
B) -megaly
C) -trophy
D) -iasis

____ **38. The suffix that means pain is**
A) -dynia
B) -penia
C) -algea
D) a and c

____ **39. The suffix -lysis means**
A) breakdown
B) destruction
C) separation
D) all of the above

____ **40. The suffix that means new opening (to form a mouth)**
A) -cut
B) -ectomy
C) -tomy
D) -ostomy

____ **41. The suffix that means little,small is**
A) -ole
B) -ule
C) -ia
D) a and b only

42. **The suffix -cyte means**
A) excision
B) cell
C) blood condition
D) pain

43. **The suffix that means resembling is**
A) -ose
B) -ous
C) -oid
D) -tic

44. **The suffix -megaly means**
A) small
B) enlarged
C) a and b
D) none of the above

45. **The suffix that means to grow**
A) -growth
B) -physis
C) -grew
D) none of the above

46. **The suffix -crine means to**
A) secrete
B) separate
C) endocrine
D) a and b only

47. **The suffix -pnea means**
A) fast
B) slow
C) breathing
D) medium

48. **The suffix -mission means to**
A) send
B) go
C) end
D) all of the above

____ 49. The suffix -lapse means to
A) slide
B) fall
C) sag
D) all of the above

____ 50. The suffix -blast means
A) to blow up
B) embryonic
C) immature
D) b and c only

____ 51. The suffix that means to birth, labor
A) -phoria
B) -partum
C) -ante
D) -post

____ 52. The suffix that means to run is
A) -run
B) -drome
C) -pour
D) -fall

____ 53. The combining form that means place, position, location is
A) top/o
B) topo
C) topo/o
D) all of the above

____ 54. The suffix that means to flow, discharge is
A) -menes
B) -rrhapy
C) -rrhea
D) -rrhexis

____ 55. The suffix that means to bear, carry
A) -burden
B) -phoria
C) -partum
D) all of the above

____ **56. The suffix that means pregnancy is**
A) -pregnat
B) -cyesis
C) -blast
D) -pregnancy

____ **57. The suffix that means above,upper is**
A) -subway
B) -supra
C) -sub
D) all of the above

Chapter 4 -The Body as a Whole

Using the list of terms below, create flash cards to learn the meaning of each prefix, prior to completing the assessment that follows.

Abdomin/o	Later/o
Adip/o	Lumb/o
Ana-	Medi/o
Anter/o	Meta-
Bol/o	Nucle/o
Cata-	-oma
Cervic/o	-ose
Chondr/o	Pelv/i
Chrom/o	-plasm
Coccyg/o	-plastic
Crani/o	Poster/o
Cyt/o	Proxim/o
Dist/o	Proxim/o
Dors/o	Sacr/o
-eal	Sarc/o
-ectomy	-some
Epi-	Spin/o
Hist/o	Thel/o
Hypo-	Thorac/o
-iac	-tomy
Ili/o	Trache/o
Inguin/o	-type
Inter-	Umbilic/o
-ior	Ventr/o
-ism	Verter/o
Kary/o	Viscer/o

Multiple Choice

Circle the most appropriate response.

____ 1. **The combining form pelv/i means**
A) hip
B) back
C) pelvic bone
D) a and c

____ 2. **The combining form that means coccyx (tailbone) is**
A) cyt/o
B) dist/o
C) coccyg/o
D) chrom/o

____ 3. **The combining form that means lower back; loin is**
A) medi/o
B) dors/o
C) lumb/o
D) poster/o

____ 4. **The combining form poster/o means**
A) after
B) from lower part of the back
C) behind
D) a and c

____ 5. **The combining form that means side is**
A) medi/o
B) anter/o
C) later/o
D) poster/o

____ 6. **The prefix that means above, upon, on is**
A) intra-
B) pro-
C) epi-
D) sub-

___ **7. The combining form hist/o means**
- A) fat
- B) nucleus
- C) organ
- D) tissue

___ **8. The combining form that means internal organs is**
- A) viscer/o
- B) sarc/o
- C) epitheli/o
- D) system/o

___ **9. The combining form thel/o means**
- A) breast
- B) nipple
- C) navel
- D) none of the above

___ **10. The suffix that means tumor; mass; fluid; collection is**
- A) -opsy
- B) -oma
- C) -cyte
- D) -al

___ **11. The combining form that means neck; cervix (neck of uterus)**
- A) neck/o
- B) cervic/o
- C) chrom/o
- D) coccyg/o

___ **12. The combining form adip/o means**
- A) fat
- B) cell
- C) tissue
- D) stomach

___ **13. The suffix -ose means**
- A) pertaining to
- B) full of
- C) sugar
- D) all of the above

____ **14. The combining form that means chest is**
A) pleur/o
B) lob/o
C) diaphragmat/o
D) thorac/o

____ **15. The combining form sacr/o means**
A) sacrum
B) flesh
C) sugar
D) none of the above

____ **16. The combining form that means front is**
A) poster/o
B) anter/o
C) abdomin/o
D) bol/o

____ **17. The combining form that means abdomen is**
A) abdomin/o
B) gastr/o
C) adip/o
D) All of the above

____ **18. The combining form spin/o means**
A) spine
B) backbone
C) flesh
D) a and b

____ **19. The combining form dist/o means movement**
A) far
B) distant
C) close
D) a and b

____ **20. The combining form umbilic/o means**
A) navel
B) stomach
C) umbilicus
D) a and c

____ 21. The suffix that means cutting into is
A) -ostomy
B) -tomy
C) a and b
D) none of the above

____ 22. The combining form that means cell is
A) cyt/o
B) eti/o
C) hist/o
D) path/o

____ 23. The combining form nucle/o means
A) neutro
B) nucleus
C) cell
D) none of the above

____ 24. The prefix that means deficient; below; under
A) trans-
B) hyper-
C) hypo-
D) pro-

____ 25. The suffix -some means
A) formation
B) picture
C) body
D) proces

____ 26. The combining form proxim/o means
A) far
B) near
C) towards
D) middle

____ 27. The combining form that means trachea (windpipe) is
A) trache/o
B) lith/o
C) son/o
D) cyst/o

____ 28. The combining form that means cartilage is
A) menisc/o
B) chondr/o
C) arthr/o
D) ten/o

____ 29. The suffix that means pertaining to is
A) -eal
B) -iac
C) -ior
D) all of the above

____ 30. The combining form chrom/o means
A) color
B) green
C) cause
D) connective tissue

____ 31. The combining form that means to cast; throw is
A) adip/o
B) cervic/o
C) chrom/o
D) bol/o

____ 32. The combining form sarc/o means
A) tumor
B) cell
C) flesh
D) cancer

____ 33. The combining form dors/o means
A) back
B) middle
C) front
D) side

____ 34. The combining form that means skull is
A) cephal/o
B) encephal/o
C) coccyg/o
D) crani/o

____ 35. The prefix that means up, apart; backward; again is
A) ab-
B) ad-
C) ante-
D) ana-

____ 36. The suffix that means formation is
A) -physis
B) -plastic
C) -plasm
D) b and c

____ 37. The combining form inguin/o means
A) stomach
B) groin
C) a and b
D) none of the above

____ 38. The combining form that means ilium (part of the pelvic bone) is
A) ili/o
B) ile/o
C) idi/o
D) all of the above

____ 39. The combining form vertebr/o means
A) chest
B) vertebra
C) backbone
D) b and c

____ 40. The prefix inter- means
A) holding
B) between
C) within
D) connecting

____ 41. The prefix that means down
A) cata-
B) contra-
C) con-
D) brady-

____ **42. The suffix -ectomy is defined as**
A) surgical repair
B) instrument used to cut
C) excision or surgical removal
D) a and c

____ **43. The combining form ventr/o means**
A) back of the body
B) middle of the body
C) side of the body
D) belly side of the body

____ **44. The combining form that means middle is**
A) medial/o
B) medi/o
C) proxim/o
D) ventr/o

____ **45. The combining form that means nucleus is**
A) umbilic/o
B) dors/o
C) inguin/o
D) kary/o

____ **46. The prefix that means change; beyond**
A) hyper-
B) neo-
C) hypo-
D) meta-

____ **47. The suffix that means process; condition is**
A) -eal
B) -ior
C) -ism
D) -ose

____ **48. The combining form that means near is**
A) dist/o
B) anter/o
C) proxim/o
D) pseud/o

____ 49. The suffix that means classification; picture
   A) -kodak
   B) -type
   C) -uria
   D) -pathy

Chapter 5-Integumentary System

Using the list of terms below, create flash cards to learn the meaning of each prefix, prior to completing the assessment that follows.

Adip/o	Myc/o
Albin/o	Onych/o
-algia	-ose
Caus/o	-osis
Cauter/o	-ous
Cutane/o	Phyt/o
Derm/o	Pil/o
-derma	-plakia
Dermat/o	-plasty
Diaphor/o	Py/o
Erythem/o	Rhytid/o
-esis	-rrhea
Hidr/o	Seb/o
Hydr/o	Sebace/o
Ichthy/o	Squam/o
Kerat/o	Steat/o
Leuk/o	Trich/o
Lip/o	Ungu/o
-lysis	Xanth/o
Melan/o	Xer/o

Multiple Choice

Circle the most appropriate response.

____ 1. **The suffix that means pain is**
   A) -cele
   B) -pexy
   C) -spasm
   D) -algia

____ 2. **The suffix that means abnormal condition is**
   A) -itis
   B) -osis
   C) -pathy
   D) -emia

____ 3. **The suffix that means surgical repair is**
   A) -angio
   B) -plasty
   C) -tomy
   D) all of the above

____ 4. **The suffix -lysis means**
   A) breakdown
   B) destruction
   C) separation
   D) all of the above

____ 5. **The suffix that means to flow, discharge is**
   A) -menes
   B) -rrhapy
   C) -rrhea
   D) -rrhexis

____ 6. **The suffix -ose means**
   A) pertaining to
   B) full of
   C) sugar
   D) all of the above

____ 7. **The suffix that means skin is**
A) -algia
B) -drama
C) -derma
D) -ose

____ 8. **The sufix that means condition is**
A) -algia
B) -derma
C) -lysis
D) -esis

____ 9. **The suffix that means pertaining to is**
A) -rrhea
B) -osis
C) -ous
D) -uos

____ 10. **The suffix -plakia means**
A) repair
B) flow
C) discharge
D) plaque

____ 11. **The combining form that means white is**
A) erythr/o
B) cyan/o
C) xanth/o
D) leuk/o

____ 12. **The combining form that means water is**
A) glyc/o
B) urin/o
C) hydr/o
D) hem/o

____ 13. **The combining form adip/o means**
A) fat
B) cell
C) tissue
D) stomach

____ **14. The combining form cutane/o means**
A) skin
B) sweat
C) oil
D) hair

____ **15. The combining form steat/o means**
A) fat
B) sugar
C) sebum
D) a and c

____ **16. The combining form lip/o mens**
A) stone
B) fat
C) liquid
D) b and c

____ **17. The combining form that means nail is**
A) ungu/o
B) onych/o
C) trich/o
D) a and b

____ **18. The combining form myc/o means**
A) fungus
B) muscle
C) oil
D) dust

____ **19. The combining form hidr/o means**
A) oil
B) sweat
C) hair
D) thick

____ **20. The combining form that means pus is**
A) pus/o
B) pus/i
C) py/o
D) py/i

____ **21. The combining form that means burn or burning is**
- A) burn/o
- B) caus/o
- C) comat/o
- D) dur/o

____ **22. The combining form albin/o means**
- A) yellow
- B) red
- C) blue
- D) white

____ **23. The combining form that means heat; burn is**
- A) heat/o
- B) red/o
- C) cauter/o
- D) all of the above

____ **24. The combining form that means skin is**
- A) derm/o
- B) dermat/o
- C) skin/o
- D) a and b

____ **25. The combining form that means sweat is**
- A) diaphor/o
- B) hydr/o
- C) seb/o
- D) all of the above

____ **26. The combining form that means flushed; redness is**
- A) erythem/o
- B) xanth/o
- C) xer/o
- D) none of the above

____ **27. The combining form ichthy/o means**
- A) dry
- B) white
- C) scaly
- D) a and c

_____ **28. The combining form kerat/o means**
   A) skin
   B) horny
   C) hard
   D) b and c

_____ **29. The combining form melan/o means**
   A) red
   B) green
   C) yellow
   D) black

_____ **30. The combining form phyt/o means**
   A) green
   B) yellow
   C) plant
   D) hair

_____ **31. The combining form that means hair is**
   A) pil/o
   B) trich/o
   C) ungu/o
   D) a and b

_____ **32. The combining form that means sebum is**
   A) py/o
   B) seb/o
   C) sebace/o
   D) b and c

_____ **33. The combining form squam/o means**
   A) acale
   B) scale
   C) sweat
   D) gland

_____ **34. The combining form xanth/o means**
   A) red
   B) green
   C) blue
   D) yellow

____ 35. The combining form that means dry is
A) hidr/o
B) xer/o
C) coni/o
D) all of the above

____ 36. The combining form that means wrinkle is
A) rrhythm/o
B) rheumat/o
C) rhin/o
D) rhytid/o

Chapter 6-Musculoskeletal System

Using the list of terms below, create flash cards to learn the meaning of each prefix, prior to completing the assessment that follows.

a-	Fibul/o	Phalang/o
Ab-	Humer/o	-physis
Acetabul/o	Humer/o	Plant/o
Ad-	Hyper-	-plasty
-algia	ili/o	Poly-
an-	Ischi/o	-porosis
Ankyl/o	Kyph/o	Pub/o
Arthr/o	kyph/o	radi/o
Arthr/o	Lamin/o	Rhabdomy/o
-asthenia	Leiomy/o	Rheumat/o
-blast	Ligament/o	Sacr/o
Burs/o	-lithesis	Sarc/o
Calc/o	Lumb/o	Scapul/o
calcen/o	-malacia	Scoli/o
Calci/o	Malleol/o	Spondyl/o
Calic/o	Mandibul/o	-stenosis
Carp/o	Maxill/o	Stern/o
Cervic/o	Meta-	sub-
Chrondr/o	-metacarp/o	Supra-
-clast	Metatars/o	Sym-
Clavicul/o	My/o	Syn-
Coccyg/o	Myos/o	Synov/o
Cost/o	Olecran/o	Tars/o
crani/o	-oma	Ten/o
-desis	Orth/o	Tendin/o
dia-	Oste/o	Thorac/o
Dorsi-	Patell/o	Tibi/o
Epi-	Ped/o	-tom
Exo-	Pelv/i	-trophy
Fasci/o	-penia	Vertebr/o
femor/o	Peri-	
Fibr/o	Perone/o	

Multiple Choice

Circle the most appropriate response.

_____ 1. **The combining form sacr/o means**
   A) sacrum
   B) flesh
   C) sugar
   D) none of the above

_____ 2. **The suffix that means nourishment, development is**
   A) -esis
   B) -megaly
   C) -trophy
   D) -iasis

_____ 3. **The combining form that means rib is**
   A) chondr/o
   B) clavic/o
   C) clavicul/o
   D) cost/o

_____ 4. **The combining form that means lower jaw bone is**
   A) mandibul/o
   B) maxill/o
   C) jaw/o
   D) odont/o

_____ 5. **The combining form stern/o means**
   A) collarbone
   B) shoulder blade
   C) xiphoid process
   D) breast bone

_____ 6. **The suffix -malacia is defined as**
   A) viewing
   B) softening
   C) eating
   D) swallowing

_____ 7. **The combining form that means muscle**
   A) mamm/o
   B) muc/o
   C) morph/o
   D) my/o

_____ 8. **The suffix -asthenia is defined as a**
   A) break
   B) split, fissure
   C) lack of strength
   D) growth

_____ 9. **The suffix -physis is defined as a**
   A) to grow
   B) break
   C) surgical fixation, fusion
   D) split, fissure

_____ 10. **The combining form rheumat/o means**
   A) joint
   B) inflammation
   C) watery flow
   D) all of the above

_____ 11. **The combining form perone/o means**
   A) fluid
   B) joint
   C) hip
   D) fibula

_____ 12. **The combining form vertebr/o means**
   A) chest
   B) vertebrae
   C) backbone
   D) b and c

_____ 13. **The combining form that means smooth muscle is**
   A) lumb/o
   B) lei/o
   C) my/o
   D) leiomy/o

____ **14. The combining form that means joint is**
A) aponeur/o
B) arthr/o
C) burs/o
D) tendin/o

____ **15. The combining form ped/o means**
A) child
B) pedicle
C) foot
D) a and c

____ **16. The suffix that means slipping is**
A) -listhesis
B) -malacia
C) -tropy
D) -tome

____ **17. The prefix that means above; upper**
A) sym-
B) supra-
C) sub-
D) poly-

____ **18. The combining form that means calcium is**
A) calc/o
B) calcane/o
C) cervic/o
D) cost/o

____ **19. The combining form that means neck; cervix (neck of uterus)**
A) neck/o
B) cervic/o
C) chrom/o
D) coccyg/o

____ **20. The suffix -clast means to**
A) break
B) bind
C) tie
D) grow

____ 21. **The combining form that means malleolus is**
A) femur/o
B) cost/o
C) my/o
D) malleol/o

____ 22. **The combining form that means hindfoot or ankle is**
A) ankl/o
B) tras/o
C) tars/o
D) all of the above

____ 23. **The combining form for bone marrow is**
A) myel/o
B) myc/o
C) myos/o
D) none of the above

____ 24. **The suffix -blast means**
A) to blow up
B) embryonic
C) immature
D) b and c only

____ 25. **The combining form that means pelvic bone (hip) is**
A) femur/o
B) hip/o
C) pelv/i
D) all of the above

____ 26. **The combining form that means humpback is**
A) kyph/o
B) ankyl/o
C) spondyl/o
D) lord/o

____ 27. **The combining form that means cartilage is**
A) menisc/o
B) chondr/o
C) arthr/o
D) ten/o

____ **28. The prefix exo- is defined as**
   A) inner
   B) around
   C) after
   D) outside

____ **29. The combining form that means sac of fluid near joints is**
   A) burss/o
   B) burs/o
   C) calc/o
   D) cost/o

____ **30. The prefix that means on, upon, over is**
   A) intra-
   B) pro-
   C) epi-
   D) sub-

____ **31. The combining form that means sole of the foot is**
   A) foot/o
   B) calcane/o
   C) tars/o
   D) plant/o

____ **32. The combining form metatars/o means**
   A) foot bones
   B) hand bones
   C) neck bones
   D) shoulder bones

____ **33. The combining form spondyl/o means**
   A) scapula
   B) vertebra
   C) cranium
   D) symphysis pubis

____ **34. The combining form ischi/o**
   A) yellowish, fatty plaque
   B) spinal cord
   C) posterior part of the pelvic bone
   D) clot

____ **35. The combining form that means fiber is**
A) fibro/o
B) fibr/o
C) fibul/o
D) humer/o

____ **36. The combining form that means kneecap is**
A) patell/o
B) phalang/o
C) rachi/o
D) orth/o

____ **37. The combining form that means striated muscle is**
A) my/o
B) cardi/o
C) rhabdomy/o
D) rhabd/o

____ **38. The prefix that means surrounding, around**
A) endo-
B) pro-
C) peri-
D) hypo-

____ **39. The combining form that means elbow is**
A) orth/o
B) humer/o
C) my/o
D) olecran/o

____ **40. The combining form that means wrist bones is**
A) carp/o
B) carp/al
C) carpal
D) all of the above

____ **41. The combining form that means bone is**
A) my/o
B) arthr/o
C) synovi/o
D) oste/o

____ **42. The combining form that means shin bone is**
   A) fibu/o
   B) humer/o
   C) radi/o
   D) tibi/o

____ **43. The combining form that means chest is**
   A) pleur/o
   B) lob/o
   C) diaphragmat/o
   D) thorac/o

____ **44. The combining form that means synovial membrane**
   A) viscer/o
   B) uln/o
   C) tars/o
   D) synov/o

____ **45. The combining form that means lower back is**
   A) medi/o
   B) dors/o
   C) lumb/o
   D) poster/o

____ **46. The combining form fibul/o means**
   A) lower arm bone
   B) uppper arm bone
   C) fibula
   D) all of the above

____ **47. The combining form that means heart muscle is**
   A) my/o
   B) cardi/o
   C) myocardi/o
   D) none of the above

____ **48. The combining form that means upper jaw bone is**
   A) madibul/o
   B) mandibul/o
   C) maxill/o
   D) myocardi/o

____ **49. The combining form scapul/o means**
A) arm
B) shoulder blade
C) ankle
D) hip

____ **50. The combining form pub/o means**
A) pelvis
B) anterior part of the hip
C) posterior part of the hip
D) none of the above

____ **51. The combining form that means fingers or toes is**
A) carp/o
B) metacarp/o
C) phalang/o
D) all of the above

____ **52. The prefix that means excessive, above**
A) hypo-
B) hyper-
C) sub-
D) trans-

____ **53. The suffix that means the instrument used to cut is**
A) -tomy
B) -ectomy
C) -ostomy
D) -tome

____ **54. The suffix that means deficiency is**
A) -algia
B) -penia
C) -sclerosis
D) -apharesis

____ **55. The combining form that means medial lower arm bone is**
A) humer/o
B) radi/o
C) uln/o
D) all of the above

____ **56. The suffix -stenosis means**
- A) tightening
- B) stricture
- C) narrowing
- D) all of the above

____ **57. The prefix for together, with is**
- A) syn-
- B) sym-
- C) growth-
- D) either a or b

____ **58. The combining form that means lamina is**
- A) lamin/o
- B) lord/o
- C) malleol/o
- D) my/o

____ **59. The prefix that means without or absence of is**
- A) a-, an-
- B) endo-
- C) intra-
- D) eu-

____ **60. The combining form radi/o means**
- A) radio
- B) radical
- C) x-rays
- D) all of the above

____ **61. The prefix that means below,under is**
- A) sub-
- B) trans-
- C) re-
- D) peri-

____ **62. The combining form that means ilium (part of the pelvic bone)**
- A) ili/o
- B) ile/o
- C) idi/o
- D) all of the above

____ **63.** **The combining form that means heel bone is**
A) calc/o
B) burs/o
C) carp/o
D) calcane/o

____ **64.** **The combining form that means curve/sway back**
A) lord/o
B) kyph/o
C) my/o
D) lumb/o

____ **65.** **The prefix that means through, complete is**
A) dia-
B) hyper-
C) dys-
D) pro-

____ **66.** **The combining form femor/o means**
A) feumr
B) femur
C) fimur
D) fimer

____ **67.** **The combining form that means skull:**
A) cephal/o
B) encephal/o
C) coccyg/o
D) crani/o

____ **68.** **The suffix -desis means to**
A) bind
B) break
C) tie together
D) a and c

____ **69.** **The prefix poly- is defined as**
A) many
B) without
C) through
D) few

____ **70. The combining form that means muscle is**
   A) orth/o
   B) arthr/o
   C) humer/o
   D) myos/o

____ **71. The suffix that means pain is**
   A) -cele
   B) -pexy
   C) -spasm
   D) -algia

____ **72. The combining form that means straight is**
   A) orth/o
   B) oste/o
   C) my/o
   D) straight/o

____ **73. The combining form sarc/o means**
   A) tumor
   B) cell
   C) flesh
   D) cancer

____ **74. The combining form acetabul/o means**
   A) ankle
   B) joint
   C) tendon
   D) acetabulum, hip socket

____ **75. The suffix that means surgical repair is**
   A) -angio
   B) -plasty
   C) -tomy
   D) all of the above

____ **76. The prefix that means toward is**
   A) an-
   B) ad-
   C) ab-
   D) ana-

____ 77. **The prefix that means away from is**
   A) a-
   B) an-
   C) ab-
   D) ad-

____ 78. **The combining form that means collar bone is**
   A) clavicul/o
   B) crani/o
   C) cost/o
   D) cervic/o

____ 79. **The suffix that means condition of the pores is**
   A) -plasty
   B) -penia
   C) -porosis
   D) -stenosis

____ 80. **The combining form metacarp/o means**
   A) hand bones
   B) foot bones
   C) shoulder
   D) knee

____ 81. **The combining form scoli/o is defined as**
   A) crooked, bent
   B) lamina
   C) stiff
   D) soft

____ 82. **The combining form that means upper arm bone is**
   A) fibul/o
   B) humer/o
   C) radi/o
   D) uln/o

____ 83. **The prefix that means after, beyond, change, is**
   A) hyper-
   B) neo-
   C) hypo-
   D) meta-

____ **84. The combining form for tendon is**
- A) ten/o
- B) tendin/o
- C) a and b
- D) none of the above

____ **85. The combining form that means fascia is**
- A) fasci/o
- B) femor/o
- C) fibr/o
- D) fibul/o

____ **86. The combining form that means joint is**
- A) arthr/o
- B) articul/o
- C) calcan/o
- D) all of the above

____ **87. The suffix that means blood condition is**
- A) -ectomy
- B) -oma
- C) -emia
- D) none of the above

____ **88. The prefix that means back is**
- A) behind-
- B) dorsi-
- C) exo-
- D) epi-

____ **89. The combining form that means ligament is**
- A) my/o
- B) maxill/o
- C) lei/o
- D) ligament/o

____ **90. The combining form ankyl/o means**
- A) stiff
- B) hump
- C) forward
- D) motion

____ **91. The combining form that means calix (calyx)**
A) calci/o
B) calic/o
C) a and b
D) none of the above

____ **92. The combining form that means tailbone is**
A) tars/o
B) carp/p
C) calcane/o
D) coccyg/o

Chapter 7-Respiratory System

Using the list of terms below, create flash cards to learn the meaning of each prefix, prior to completing the assessment that follows.

A-
Adenoid/o
-algia
-algia
Alveol/o
An-
Brady-
Bronch/o
Bronchi/o
Capn/o
-capnia
-centesis
Coni/o
Cyan/o
-dynia
Dys-
-ectasis
-ectomy
Em-
Epiglott/o
Eu-
Ex-
Hydr/o
Hyper/o
Hypo-
Laryng/o
Lob/o
-lysis
Mediastin/o
Nas/o
Or/o
Orth/o
-osmia
-ostomy
Ox/o

-oxia
Para-
Pector/o
Per-
Pharyng/o
Phon/o
-phonia
Phren/o
-plasty
Pleur/o
-pnea
Pneumon/o
Pneumon/o
-ptysis
Pulmon/o
Pulmon/o
Py/o
Re-
Rhin/o
-rrhea
-scopy
Sinus/o
-sphyxia
Spir/o
-stenosis
Stomat/o
Tachy-
Tel/o
Thorac/o
-thorax
-tomy
Tonsil/o
Trache/o
-trophy

Multiple Choice

Circle the most appropriate response.

____ 1. **The suffix that means surgical puncture to aspirate fluid is**
   A) -capnia
   B) -centesis
   C) -tomy
   D) -either b or c

____ 2. **The suffix -stenosis means**
   A) tightening
   B) stricture
   C) narrowing
   D) all of the above

____ 3. **The combining form that means diaphragm is**
   A) -phreno
   B) phren/o
   C) par/o
   D) ox/o

____ 4. **The combining form that means throat is**
   A) pharyng/o
   B) throat/o
   C) stomat/o
   D) somat/o

____ 5. **The combining form that means dust is**
   A) coni/o
   B) necr/o
   C) myc/o
   D) crypt/o

____ 6. **The combining form ox/o means**
   A) carbon dioxide
   B) oxen
   C) oxygen
   D) infections

____ 7. **The suffix -ectomy is defined as**
A) surgical repair
B) instrument used to cut
C) excision or surgical removal
D) a and c

____ 8. **The prefix that means near; beside**
A) neo-
B) para-
C) per-
D) meta-

____ 9. **The combining form that means membrane surrounding the lungs is**
A) dur/o
B) pleur/o
C) lung/o
D) pneumon/o

____ 10. **The prefix that means without or absence of is**
A) a, an-
B) endo-
C) intra-
D) eu-

____ 11. **The combining form that means water is**
A) glyc/o
B) urin/o
C) hydr/o
D) hem/o

____ 12. **The combining form that means carbon dioxide is**
A) cardi/o
B) capn/o
C) cac/o
D) CO2

____ 13. **The suffix that means voice; sound**
A) -phoria
B) -phonia
C) -phagia
D) all of the above

____ 14. **The combining form tonsil/o means**
   A) tonsils
   B) tonsillitis
   C) tonsills
   D) none of the above

____ 15. **The combining form that means lung is**
   A) pulmon/o
   B) pneumon/o
   C) broncho
   D) a and b

____ 16. **The combining form that means blue is**
   A) erythr/o
   B) leuk/o
   C) xanth/o
   D) cyan/o

____ 17. **The suffix that means chest; pleural cavity**
   A) -tharox
   B) -thorax
   C) -tomy
   D) -tachy

____ 18. **The prefix that means good, normal**
   A) normo-
   B) eu-
   C) ex-
   D) brady-

____ 19. **The suffix that means repair is**
   A) -angio
   B) -plasty
   C) -tomy
   D) all of the above

____ 20. **The suffix that means the process of cutting**
   A) -ostomy
   B) -tomy
   C) -ology
   D) -scopy

____ **21. The combining form that means nose**
   A) rhin/a
   B) nas/o
   C) or/o
   D) tel/o

____ **22. The suffix that means pain is**
   A) -dynia
   B) -penia
   C) -algia
   D) a and c

____ **23. The suffix -lysis means**
   A) breakdown
   B) destruction
   C) separation
   D) all of the above

____ **24. The prefix that means slow**
   A) bi-
   B) brady-
   C) con-
   D) contra-

____ **25. The combining form epiglott/o means**
   A) throat
   B) windpipe
   C) epiglottis
   D) all of the above

____ **26. The combining form that means breathe, breathing is**
   A) atel/o
   B) ox/o
   C) spir/o
   D) pneum/o

____ **27. The combining form that means pus is**
   A) pyr/o
   B) pyel/o
   C) py/o
   D) pus/o

____ **28. The prefix that means above; excessive**
- A) hypo-
- B) hyper-
- C) sub-
- D) trans-

____ **29. The combining form for mouth is**
- A) stomat/o
- B) or/o
- C) esophag/o
- D) a and b

____ **30. The suffix that means spitting is**
- A) -ptysis
- B) -ptosis
- C) -plasty
- D) -phagia

____ **31. The suffix that means pain is**
- A) -cele
- B) -pexy
- C) -spasm
- D) -algia

____ **32. The prefix that means out is**
- A) ex-
- B) epi-
- C) endo-
- D) a and b

____ **33. The suffix -osmia means**
- A) oxygen
- B) carbon dioxide
- C) chloride
- D) smell

____ **34. The combining form phon/o means**
- A) pus
- B) voice
- C) sound
- D) b and c

____ **35. The prefix that means fast, rapid is**
A) brady-
B) tachy-
C) hyper-
D) meta-

____ **36. The combining form that means lung is**
A) pulmon/o
B) pneumon/o
C) broncho
D) a and b

____ **37. The prefix re- means**
A) back
B) backward
C) again
D) all of the above

____ **38. The combining form that means trachea (windpipe) is**
A) trache/o
B) lith/o
C) son/o
D) cyst/o

____ **39. The combining form alveol/o means**
A) alveolus
B) air sac
C) small sac
D) all of the above

____ **40. The combining form that means bronchiole is**
A) bronch/o
B) bronchi/o
C) bronchiol/o
D) all of the above

____ **41. The suffix -oxia means**
A) carbon dioxide
B) H2O
C) oxygen
D) sugar

____ **42. The prefix dys- means**
   A) bad, painful
   B) difficult, abnormal
   C) a and b
   D) none of the above

____ **43. The combining form that means sinus is**
   A) steth/o
   B) sinus/o
   C) senus/o
   D) all of the above

____ **44. The suffix -pnea means**
   A) fast
   B) slow
   C) breathing
   D) medium

____ **45. The combining form lob/o means**
   A) lung
   B) lobe
   C) tube
   D) all of the above

____ **46. The combining form orth/o means**
   A) straight
   B) oxygen
   C) incomplete
   D) breathe

____ **47. The prefix that means through**
   A) per-
   B) peri-
   C) transit-
   D) poly-

____ **48. The combining form mediastin/o means**
   A) chest
   B) stomach
   C) mediastinem
   D) mediastinum

____ 49. The combining form that means chest is
- A) pleur/o
- B) lob/o
- C) diaphragmat/o
- D) thorac/o

____ 50. The combining form that means bronchial tubes is
- A) pulmon/o
- B) bronchi/o
- C) bronch/o
- D) b and c

____ 51. The combining form that means adenoids is
- A) aden/o
- B) adenoid/o
- C) a and b
- D) none of the above

____ 52. The prefix em- means
- A) impossible
- B) important
- C) emesis
- D) in

____ 53. The combining form that means chest is
- A) patella
- B) tel/o
- C) phon/o
- D) pector/o

____ 54. The suffix that means pulse is
- A) -thorax
- B) -oxia
- C) -phonia
- D) -sphyxia

____ 55. The combining form rhin/o means
- A) nose
- B) sinus
- C) septum
- D) air

____ **56. The suffix that means new opening (to form a mouth)**
   A) -cut
   B) -ectomy
   C) -tomy
   D) -ostomy

____ **57. The combining form tel/o means**
   A) telephone
   B) distant
   C) near
   D) complete

____ **58. The suffix meaning stretching;dilation; expansion is**
   A) -ectasis
   B) -centesis
   C) -capnia
   D) -pnea

____ **59. The suffix that means carbon dioxide is**
   A) -CO2
   B) -capnia
   C) -captain
   D) none of the above

____ **60. The suffix that means the process of viewing**
   A) -scopy
   B) -scope
   C) -gram
   D) -graphy

____ **61. The combining form that means voice box is**
   A) larynx
   B) laryng/o
   C) lymph/o
   D) lapar/o

____ **62. The prefix that means deficient; below; under**
   A) trans-
   B) hyper-
   C) hypo-
   D) pro-

____ **63. The suffix that means nourishment, development is**
- A) -esis
- B) -megaly
- C) -trophy
- D) -iasis

____ **64. The suffix that means to flow, discharge is**
- A) -menes
- B) -rrhapy
- C) -rrhea
- D) -rrhexis

Chapter 8-Cardiovascular System

Using the list of terms below, create flash cards to learn the meaning of each prefix, prior to completing the assessment that follows.

a-	-megaly
an-	-meter
Aneurysm/o	My/o
Angi/o	Myx/o
Aort/o	-oma
Arteri/o	-osis
Ather/o	Ox/o
Atri/o	Percardi/o
Axill/o	Peri-
Brachi/o	Phleb/o
Brady-	-plasty
Cardi/o	Pulmon/o
Cholesterol/o	-sclerosis
-constriction	Sphygm/o
Coron/o	Steth/o
Cyan/o	Tachy-
de-	Tetra-
-dilation	Thromb/o
Dys-	-tomy
-emia	Tri-
Endo-	Valv/o
-graphy	Valvul/o
Hyper-	Vas/o
Hypo-	vascul/o
Inter-	Ven/i
Isch/o	Ven/o
-lysis	Ventricul/o

Multiple Choice

Circle the most appropriate response.

____ 1. **The combining form angi/o means**
   A) vessel
   B) duct
   C) vein
   D) none of the above

____ 2. **The suffix that means the process of recording**
   A) -gram
   B) -graph
   C) -grahpy
   D) -all of the above

____ 3. **The combining form that means vessel; duct; vas deferens is**
   A) valv/o
   B) ven/o
   C) vas/o
   D) vaso

____ 4. **The prefix that means above; excessive**
   A) hypo-
   B) hyper-
   C) sub-
   D) trans-

____ 5. **The prefix that means four**
   A) trio-
   B) tri-
   C) tetra-
   D) all of the above

____ 6. **The suffix -megaly means**
   A) small
   B) enlarged
   C) a and b
   D) none of the above

____ 7. **The prefix that means in; within**
A) uni-
B) retro-
C) ante-
D) endo-

____ 8. **The combining form isch/o means**
A) yellowish, fatty plaque
B) sound
C) to hold back
D) clot

____ 9. **The combining form the means blue**
A) erythr/o
B) leuk/o
C) xanth/o
D) cyan/o

____ 10. **The suffix -dilation means to**
A) widening
B) stretching
C) expanding
D) all of the above

____ 11. **The combining form that means mucus is**
A) my/o
B) myel/o
C) myc/o
D) myx/o

____ 12. **The prefix that means fast, rapid is**
A) brady-
B) tachy-
C) hyper-
D) meta-

____ 13. **The suffix that means tumor is**
A) -opsy
B) -oma
C) -cyte
D) -al

_____ **14.** **The combining form that means atrium (upper heart chamber) is**
A) atri/o
B) aut/o
C) aort/o
D) ven/o

_____ **15.** **The prefix dys- means**
A) bad, painful
B) difficult, abnormal
C) a and b
D) none of the above

_____ **16.** **The combining form aneurysm/o means**
A) aneurysm
B) vechile
C) clumping
D) to assemble, gather

_____ **17.** **The combining form pericardi/o means**
A) heart
B) around
C) surrounding the heart
D) none of the above

_____ **18.** **The combining form cholesterol/o means**
A) sugar
B) fat
C) amino acid
D) cholesterol

_____ **19.** **The combining form that means muscle is**
A) mamm/o
B) muc/o
C) morph/o
D) my/o

_____ **20.** **The combining form that means vein is**
A) ven/o
B) ven/i
C) phleb/o
D) all of the above

____ **21. The combining form that means arm is**
   A) brachi/o
   B) bronch/o
   C) brach/o
   D) bilirubin/o

____ **22. The combining form that means oxygen is**
   A) ox/o
   B) ooxy/o
   C) ox/oo
   D) all of the above

____ **23. The prefix that means surrounding,around**
   A) endo-
   B) pro-
   C) peri-
   D) hypo-

____ **24. The combining form that means lung is**
   A) pulmon/o
   B) steth/o
   C) a and b
   D) none of the above

____ **25. The combining form that means armpit is**
   A) armpit/o
   B) axilll/o
   C) axill/o
   D) azot/o

____ **26. The suffix -stenosis means**
   A) tightening
   B) stricture
   C) narrowing
   D) all of the above

____ **27. The combining form that means valve is**
   A) valv/o
   B) valvul/o
   C) ventricul/o
   D) a and b

____ **28. The suffix -constriction means**
A) narrowing
B) construct
C) construction
D) close

____ **29. The prefix that means slow**
A) bi-
B) brady-
C) con-
D) contra-

____ **30. The prefix inter- means**
A) holding
B) between
C) within
D) connecting

____ **31. The suffix that means repair is**
A) -angio
B) -plasty
C) -tomy
D) all of the above

____ **32. The combining form that means artery is**
A) arti/o
B) aort/o
C) angi/o
D) arteri/o

____ **33. The suffix that means hardening is**
A) -malacia
B) -sclerosis
C) -penia
D) -crit

____ **34. The combining form that means heart is**
A) atri/o
B) phleb/o
C) ventricul/o
D) coron/o

____ 35. The suffix that means abnormal condition is
A) -itis
B) -osis
C) -pathy
D) -emia

____ 36. The combining form sphygm/o means
A) pulse
B) chest
C) sound
D) a and c

____ 37. The prefix that means three
A) tri-
B) quadri-
C) tetra-
D) bi-

____ 38. The combining form ather/o means
A) fatty substance
B) plaque
C) atrium
D) a and b

____ 39. The combining form cardi/o means
A) lung
B) liver
C) cards
D) heart

____ 40. The prefix that means deficient; below; under
A) trans-
B) hyper-
C) hypo-
D) pro-

____ 41. The suffix -meter means to
A) make
B) measure
C) view
D) take

____ 42. The combining form that means ventricle is
A) atri/o
B) aort/o
C) ather/o
D) ventricul/o

____ 43. The suffix that means the process of cutting
A) -ostomy
B) -tomy
C) -ology
D) -scopy

____ 44. The combining form aort/o means
A) white
B) pain
C) aorta
D) ulcer

____ 45. The combining form thromb/o means
A) sound
B) heat
C) electricity
D) clot

____ 46. The suffix that means blood condition is
A) -ectomy
B) -oma
C) -emia
D) none of the above

____ 47. The combining form that means chest is
A) pleur/o
B) lob/o
C) diaphragmat/o
D) steth/o

____ 48. The suffix -lysis means
A) breakdown
B) destruction
C) separation
D) all of the above

____ **49. The prefix that means without or absence of is**
   A) a, an-
   B) endo-
   C) intra-
   D) eu-

____ **50. The prefix de- means**
   A) down
   B) up
   C) lack of
   D) a and c

____ **51. The combining form that means vessel; duct; vas deferens**
   A) ven/o
   B) ven/i
   C) vavl/o
   D) vascul/o

Chapter 9-Lymphatic System

Using the list of terms below, create flash cards to learn the meaning of each prefix, prior to completing the assessment that follows.

Ana-
Auto-
Axill/o
Cervic/o
-cytosis
-edema
-globin
-globulin
Hyper-
Immun/o
Inguin/o
Inter-
Lymph/o
Lymphaden/o
-megaly
-oid
-pathy
-penia
-phylaxis
-poiesis
Retro-
Splen/o
-stitial
-suppression
Thym/o
Tox/o

Multiple Choice

Circle the most appropriate response.

____ 1. **The combining form that means armpit is**
A) axill/o
B) axilla
C) armpit/o
D) none of the above

____ 2. **The combining form inguin/o means**
A) stomach
B) groin
C) a and b
D) none of the above

____ 3. **The combining form that means neck; cervix (neck of uterus)**
A) neck/o
B) cervic/o
C) chrom/o
D) coccyg/o

____ 4. **The combining form lymphaden/o means**
A) spleen
B) thymus gland
C) lymph gland
D) all of the above

____ 5. **The combining form that means thymus gland is**
A) lyphaden/o
B) splen/o
C) thymo/o
D) thym/o

____ 6. **The combining form that means protection;safe is**
A) immunit/o
B) immune/o
C) immun/o
D) all of the above

____ 7. **The combining form that means spleen is**
A) chole/o
B) spleno/o
C) splen/o
D) b and c

____ 8. **The combining form that means poison is**
A) kal/i
B) acr/o
C) tox/o
D) calc/i

____ 9. **The combining form that means lymph**
A) lymph
B) lymph/o
C) a and b
D) b and c

____ 10. **The prefix inter- means**
A) holding
B) between
C) within
D) connecting

____ 11. **The prefix retro- means**
A) back
B) backward
C) behind
D) all of the above

____ 12. **The prefix that means up, apart is**
A) ab-
B) ad-
C) ante-
D) ana-

____ 13. **The prefix that means self is**
A) bi-
B) auto-
C) hetero-
D) none of the above

____ **14. The prefix that means excessive, above**
A) hypo-
B) hyper-
C) sub-
D) trans-

____ **15. The suffix that means to stop**
A) -retro
B) -suppression
C) -inter
D) -oid

____ **16. The suffix -cytosis means**
A) condition of cells
B) slight increase in the number of cells
C) cell
D) a and b

____ **17. The suffix that means disease**
A) -ology
B) -pathy
C) -tomy
D) -ion

____ **18. The suffix that means swelling is**
A) -cytosis
B) -edema
C) -oid
D) -megaly

____ **19. The suffix -megaly means**
A) small
B) enlargement
C) a and b
D) none of the above

____ **20. The suffix -poiesis means**
A) removal
B) separation
C) hardening
D) formation

____ **21. The suffix that means deficiency is**
     A) -algia
     B) -penia
     C) -sclerosis
     D) -apharesis

____ **22. The suffix that means protein is**
     A) -globin
     B) -globulin
     C) -prote
     D) a and b

____ **23. The suffix that means to set is**
     A) -suppression
     B) -penia
     C) -stitial
     D) -set

____ **24. The suffix that means protection is**
     A) -plasia
     B) -poiesis
     C) -phylaxis
     D) -suppression

____ **25. The suffix that means resembling**
     A) -ose
     B) -ous
     C) -oid
     D) -tic

Chapter 10-Blood

Using the list of terms below, create flash cards to learn the meaning of each prefix, prior to completing the assessment that follows.

a-	Mega-
an-	Micro-
Anti-	Mon/o
-apheresis	Mono-
Bas/o	Morph/o
-blast	Myel/o
Chrom/o	Neutr/o
Coagul/o	Nucle/o
Cyt/o	-oid
-cytosis	-osis
-emia	Pan-
Eosin/o	-penia
Erythr/o	Phag/o
-globin	-phage
-globulin	-philia
Granul/o	-phoresis
Hem/o	-plasia
Hemat/o	-poiesis
Hemoglobin/o	Poikil/o
Hypo-	Poly-
Is/o	Sider/o
Kary/o	Sper/o
Leuk/o	-stasis
-lytic	Thromb/o

Multiple Choice

Circle the most appropriate response.

____ 1. **The combining form that means white**
   A) erythr/o
   B) cyan/o
   C) xanth/o
   D) leuk/o

____ 2. **The combining form hem/o, hemat/o means**
   A) hemoglobin
   B) hematocrit
   C) blood
   D) plasma

____ 3. **The combining form that means coagulation is**
   A) coagul/o
   B) hem/o
   C) hemat/o
   D) all of the above

____ 4. **The combining form that means nucleus**
   A) umbilic/o
   B) dors/o
   C) inguin/o
   D) kary/o

____ 5. **The combining form that means iron is**
   A) iron/o
   B) sider/o
   C) spher/o
   D) all of the above

____ 6. **The combining form myel/o is defined as**
   A) spinal cord
   B) gray matter
   C) brain
   D) nerve root

____ 7. **The combining form that means red is**
- A) xanth/o
- B) leuk/o
- C) erythr/o
- D) melan/o

____ 8. **The combining form that means cell is**
- A) cyt/o
- B) eti/o
- C) hist/o
- D) path/o

____ 9. **The combining form that means red rosy; dawn colored**
- A) bas/o
- B) eosin/o
- C) hem/o
- D) all of the above

____ 10. **The combining form that means to eat;swallow**
- A) eat/o
- B) ate/o
- C) phag/o
- D) sider/o

____ 11. **The combining form that means same;equal**
- A) isi/o
- B) is/o
- C) sam/o
- D) equ/o

____ 12. **The combining form that means hemoglobin**
- A) hem/o
- B) globin/o
- C) hemoglobin/o
- D) a and b

____ 13. **The combining form neutr/o means**
- A) neutron
- B) neutrophil
- C) neutral, neither
- D) nucleus

____ **14. The combining form chrom/o is defined as**
- A) color
- B) green
- C) cause
- D) connective tissue

____ **15. The combining form that means shape; form**
- A) muc/o
- B) morph/o
- C) my/o
- D) myel/o

____ **16. The combining for that means granule**
- A) gran/o
- B) granul/o
- C) hem/o
- D) hemat/o

____ **17. The combining form bas/o means**
- A) basic
- B) base
- C) opposite of acid
- D) b and c

____ **18. The combining form that means one;single**
- A) tri/o
- B) tetr/o
- C) mon/o
- D) all of the above

____ **19. The combining form that means varied; irregular**
- A) phag/o
- B) poikil/o
- C) sider/o
- D) spher/o

____ **20. The combining form thromb/o is defined as**
- A) sound
- B) heat
- C) electricity
- D) clot

____ 21. The combining form nucle/o means
A) neutro
B) nucleus
C) nucleo
D) none of the above

____ 22. The combining form that means round; globe shaped
A) sper/o
B) spher/o
C) sider/o
D) all of the above

____ 23. The prefix that means deficient, below, under
A) trans-
B) hyper-
C) hypo-
D) pro-

____ 24. The prefix mega- means
A) small
B) large
C) enlarged
D) many

____ 25. The prefix that means one;single is
A) tri-
B) tetra-
C) poly-
D) mono-

____ 26. The prefix that means large
A) macro-
B) mal-
C) hemi-
D) meta-

____ 27. The prefix that means small is
A) nulli-
B) macro-
C) multi-
D) micro-

28. The prefix that means against is
   A) ante-
   B) anti-
   C) auto-
   D) cata-

29. The prefix poly- is defined as
   A) many
   B) without
   C) through
   D) few

30. The prefix that means all
   A) peri-
   B) pan-
   C) per-
   D) para-

31. The prefix that means without or absence of is
   A) a-, an-
   B) endo-
   C) intra-
   D) eu-

32. The suffix -cytosis means
   A) condition of cells
   B) slight increase in the number of cells
   C) cell
   D) a and b

33. The suffix that means removal is
   A) -phage
   B) -stasis
   C) -blast
   D) -apheresis

34. The suffix -blast means
   A) to blow up
   B) embryonic
   C) immature
   D) b and c only

____ **35. The suffix that means control, stop, standing is**
   A) -osis
   B) -plasm
   C) -genesis
   D) -stasis

____ **36. The suffix -poiesis means**
   A) removal
   B) separation
   C) hardening
   D) formation

____ **37. The suffix that means deficiency is**
   A) -algia
   B) -penia
   C) -sclerosis
   D) -apharesis

____ **38. The suffix that means eat; swallow**
   A) -philia
   B) -plasia
   C) -phage
   D) none of the above

____ **39. The suffix -philia means**
   A) attraction for
   B) small
   C) blood
   D) stop

____ **40. The suffix that means to reduce, destroy**
   A) -less
   B) -lytic
   C) -letgo
   D) none of the above

____ **41. The suffix that means blood condition is**
   A) -ectomy
   B) -oma
   C) -emia
   D) none of the above

____ **42. The suffix -plasia is defined as**
   A) formation, development, growth
   B) causing
   C) substance or agent
   D) abnormal condition

____ **43. The suffix that means carrying; transmission**
   A) -plasia
   B) -phoresis
   C) -poiesis
   D) -oid

____ **44. The suffix that means resembling**
   A) -ose
   B) -ous
   C) -oid
   D) -tic

____ **45. The suffix that means protein is**
   A) -globin
   B) -globulin
   C) -gen
   D) a and b

____ **46. The suffix that means condition is**
   A) -oid
   B) -opsy
   C) -osis
   D) -tic

Chapter 11-Digestive System

Using the list of terms below, create flash cards to learn the meaning of each prefix, prior to completing the assessment that follows.

Amyl/o	Eti/o	-ostomy
An/o	Gastr/o	Palat/o
Append/o	-genesis	Pancreat/o
Appendic/o	Gingiv/o	-pathy
-ase	Gloss/o	-pepsia
Bil/i	Gluc/o	Peritone/o
Bilirubin/o	Glycogen/o	-phagia
Bronch/o	-graphy	Pharyng/o
Bucc/o	Gylc/o	-plasty
Cec/o	Hem/o	-prandial
Celi/o	Hemat/o	Proct/o
-centesis	Hepat/o	Prote/o
Cervic/o	Herni/o	-ptosis
Cheil/o	-iasis	-ptysis
-chezia	Idi/o	Pylor/o
Chlorhydr/o	Ile/o	Rect/o
Chol/e	Jejun/o	-rrhage
Cholangi/o	Labi/o	-rrhagia
Cholecyst/o	Lapar/o	-rrhaphy
Choledoch/o	Lingu/o	-rrhea
Cib/o	Lip/o	-scopy
Cirrh/o	Lith/o	Sialaden/o
Col/o	Lymphangi/o	Sigmoid/o
Dent/i	-lysis	-spasm
Duoden/o	Mandibul/o	Spleen/o
-ectasis	-megaly	-stasis
-ectasis	Men/o	Steat/o
-ectomy	Necr/o	-stenosis
-emesis	Odyn/o	Stomat/o
-emia	Ondont/o	-tomy
Enter/o	Or/o	Tonsill/o
Esophag/o	-orexia	-tresia

Multiple Choice

Circle the most appropriate response.

____ 1. **The suffix that means new opening**
   A) -ectomy
   B) -ostomy
   C) -tomy
   D) -sthenia

____ 2. **The combining form that means appendix is**
   A) append/o
   B) appendic/o
   C) bucc/o
   D) a and b

____ 3. **The combining form that means salivary gland is**
   A) sialadeno
   B) sialaden/o
   C) sigmoid/o
   D) none of the above

____ 4. **The combining form herni/o means**
   A) hernia
   B) umbilicus
   C) ventral
   D) anterior

____ 5. **The combining form bil/i means**
   A) gall
   B) bile
   C) ball
   D) a and b

____ 6. **The combining form glycogen/o means**
   A) animal starch
   B) glycogen
   C) a and b
   D) none of the above

____ 7. The combining form that means pain is

   A) pain/o
   B) odont/o
   C) odyn/o
   D) ocul/o

____ 8. The combining form that means tongue is

   A) labi/o
   B) lingu/o
   C) tong/o
   D) glos/o

____ 9. The combining form cec/o means

   A) colon
   B) appendix
   C) ileum
   D) cecum

____ 10. The suffix that means blood condition is

   A) -ectomy
   B) -oma
   C) -emia
   D) none of the above

____ 11. The combining form lymphangi/o means

   A) lymph
   B) lymph vessel
   C) vessel
   D) none of the above

____ 12. The combining form steat/o means

   A) fat
   B) sugar
   C) sebum
   D) a and c

____ 13. The combining form for rectum is

   A) par/o
   B) ped/o
   C) rect/o
   D) a and c

____ **14. The combining form for gall, bile is**
A) cheil/o
B) choledoch/o
C) chol/e
D) cholangi/o

____ **15. The suffix -lysis means**
A) breakdown
B) destruction
C) separation
D) all of the above

____ **16. The combining form that means pancreas is**
A) palat/o
B) pancreat/o
C) peritone/o
D) pancre/o

____ **17. The suffix -prandial means**
A) stone
B) gall
C) prandial
D) meal

____ **18. The suffix that means appetite**
A) -orexia
B) -prandial
C) -cibo
D) -oid

____ **19. The combining form that means tooth is**
A) odont/o
B) lingu/o
C) tooth/o
D) teeth/o

____ **20. The combining form that means tongue is**
A) tongu/o
B) tongue
C) gloss/o
D) glosso

____ 21. The suffix that means control, stop, standing is
A) -osis
B) -plasm
C) -genesis
D) -stasis

____ 22. The combining form hem/o, hemat/o means
A) hemoglobin
B) hematocrit
C) blood
D) plasma

____ 23. The combining form chlorhydr/o means
A) chloride
B) hydrochloride
C) hydrochloric acid
D) none of the above

____ 24. The combining form men/o is defined as
A) last, ending
B) menstruation
C) first, beginning
D) regular

____ 25. The combining form for intestines (usually the small intestine) is
A) col/o
B) or/o
C) ile/o
D) enter/o

____ 26. The combining form bronch/o means
A) bronchial tube
B) tube
C) bronchial
D) none of the above

____ 27. The combining form that means duodenum
A) douden/a
B) duoden/a
C) douden/o
D) duoden/o

____ 28. The combining form that means throat

A) pharyng/o
B) throat/o
C) stomat/o
D) somat/o

____ 29. The combining form gluc/o means

A) glucus
B) sugar
C) fat
D) protein

____ 30. The combining form that means spleen is

A) chole/o
B) spleno/o
C) splen/o
D) b and c

____ 31. The combining form tonsill/o means

A) tonsils
B) tonsillitis
C) tonsills
D) none of the above

____ 32. The combining that means ileum is

A) ile/o
B) ili/o
C) a and b
D) none of the above

____ 33. The combining form that means meals is

A) meal/o
B) ant/o
C) cib/o
D) none of the above

____ 34. The suffix that means repair is

A) -angio
B) -plasty
C) -tomy
D) all of the above

_____ 35. The combining form cholangi/o means
A) bile vessel
B) gall bladder
C) relaxation
D) drug

_____ 36. The combining form that means stone or calculus is
A) blast/o
B) lith/o
C) tom/o
D) azot/o

_____ 37. The combining form sigmoid/o means
A) meat
B) sigmoid colon
C) body
D) stomat

_____ 38. The combining form idi/o means
A) idiot
B) unknown
C) individual
D) b and c

_____ 39. The suffix -iasis means
A) abormal condition
B) pancreas
C) meal
D) none of the above

_____ 40. The combining form that means palate is
A) palat/o
B) plata/o
C) palata/o
D) polat/o

_____ 41. The combining form that means pyloric sphincter is
A) polyp/o
B) proct/o
C) rect/o
D) pylor/o

____ **42. The suffix that means cutting into is**
A) -ostomy
B) -tomy
C) a and b
D) none of the above

____ **43. The suffix that means to flow, discharge is**
A) -menes
B) -rrhapy
C) -rrhea
D) -rrhexis

____ **44. The combining form lapar/o means**
A) pelvis
B) abdominal wall
C) laparum
D) none of the above

____ **45. The combining form for mouth is**
A) stomat/o
B) or/o
C) esophag/o
D) a and b

____ **46. The combining form that means peritoneum**
A) peritoneum/o
B) perit/o
C) peritone/o
D) periton/o

____ **47. The combining form that means cause of disease is**
A) melan/o
B) path/o
C) carcin/o
D) eti/o

____ **48. The combining form that means gallbadder is**
A) celi/o
B) cheil/o
C) cholecyst/o
D) all of the above

____ **49. The suffix -ptosis means**
A) drooping
B) sagging
C) proplase
D) all of the above

____ **50. The suffix -pepsia means**
A) opening
B) small growth
C) tumor
D) digestion

____ **51. The suffix that means surgical puncture to aspirate fluid is**
A) -capnia
B) -centesis
C) -tomy
D) -either b or c

____ **52. The suffix that means sudden, involuntary contraction of muscles:**
A) -stasis
B) -spasm
C) -ptosis
D) -lysis

____ **53. The combing form that means gums is**
A) gum/o
B) gloss/o
C) gastr/o
D) gingiv/o

____ **54. The suffix -ase means**
A) sugar
B) meal
C) enzyme
D) gall

____ **55. The combining form cirrh/o means**
A) red
B) green
C) orange-yellow
D) white

____ **56. The combining form for liver is**
A) hepat/o
B) lingu/o
C) palat/o
D) uvul/o

____ **57. The suffix that means suturing, repairing is**
A) -megaly
B) -trophy
C) -rrhaphy
D) -esis

____ **58. The suffix that means spitting is**
A) -ptysis
B) -ptosis
C) -plasty
D) -phagia

____ **59. The suffix that means the process of recording**
A) -gram
B) -graph
C) -grahpy
D) -all of the above

____ **60. The combining form that means cheek is**
A) cheek/o
B) bucc/o
C) cec/o
D) celi/o

____ **61. The combining form that means lower jaw bone is**
A) mandibul/o
B) maxill/o
C) jaw/o
D) odont/o

____ **62. The combining form that means lip is**
A) ex/o
B) lip/o
C) labi/o
D) odont/o

____ **63. The suffix -megaly means**
- A) small
- B) enlargement
- C) a and b
- D) none of the above

____ **64. The suffix that means streching, dilation, expansion**
- A) -lysis
- B) -emesis
- C) -ectasia
- D) -pepsia

____ **65. The combining form that means death is**
- A) necr/o
- B) pachy/o
- C) coni/o
- D) aut/o

____ **66. The combining form that means tooth**
- A) tooth/o
- B) dent/i
- C) a and b
- D) none of the above

____ **67. The combining form bilirubin/o means**
- A) bile pigment
- B) bilirubin
- C) increase
- D) a and b

____ **68. The combining form that means common bile duct is**
- A) cholecyst/o
- B) choledoch/o
- C) colon/o
- D) a and b

____ **69. The suffix that means bursting forth of blood is:**
- A) -rrhagia
- B) -rrhage
- C) -rrhaphy
- D) a and b

____ **70. The suffix -phagia is defined as**
A) surgical repair
B) softening
C) disease or abnormal state
D) eating or swallowing

____ **71. The combining form lip/o mens**
A) stone
B) fat
C) lipid
D) b and c

____ **72. The suffix that means the process of viewing**
A) -scopy
B) -scope
C) -gram
D) -graphy

____ **73. The combining form that means sugar is**
A) hidr/o
B) hydr/o
C) glyc/o
D) a and c

____ **74. The combining form that means anus is**
A) bucc/o
B) cec/o
C) append/o
D) an/o

____ **75. The combining form that means jejunum is**
A) jejum/o
B) jejun/o
C) a and b
D) none of the above

____ **76. The suffix that means producing;forming is**
A) -genesis
B) -ous
C) -gentle
D) a and c

____ 77. The combining form cheil/o means
A) gall, bile
B) lip
C) tongue
D) saliva

____ 78. The combining form that means neck; cervix (neck of uterus) is
A) neck/o
B) cervic/o
C) chrom/o
D) coccyg/o

____ 79. The suffix -stenosis means
A) tightening
B) stricture
C) narrowing
D) all of the above

____ 80. The combining form prote/o means
A) fat
B) sugar
C) protein
D) stone

____ 81. The suffix -chezia means
A) elimination
B) defecation
C) meal
D) a and b

____ 82. The suffix that means opening is
A) -stenosis
B) -spasm
C) -tresia
D) -pepsia

____ 83. The combining form that means stomach is
A) somat/o
B) stomat/o
C) hepat/o
D) gastr/o

____ **84. The combining form that means colon is**
   A) col/o
   B) colon/o
   C) colo/o
   D) a and b

____ **85. The suffix that means disease**
   A) -ology
   B) -pathy
   C) -tomy
   D) -ion

____ **86. The suffix that means stretching; dilation; expansion is**
   A) -ectasis
   B) -centesis
   C) -capnia
   D) -pnea

____ **87. The combining form that means esophagus is**
   A) esophag/o
   B) eophag/o
   C) a and b
   D) none of the above

____ **88. The combining form amyl/o means**
   A) gall
   B) amylus
   C) starch
   D) fat

____ **89. The combining form proct/o means**
   A) anus
   B) rectum
   C) pancreas
   D) a and b

____ **90. The suffix that means vomiting**
   A) -ectasia
   B) -ectasis
   C) -emesis
   D) -phagia

____ 91. The combining form celi/o means
- A) abdomen
- B) stomach
- C) lip
- D) mouth

____ 92. The suffix -ectomy is defined as
- A) surgical repair
- B) instrument used to cut
- C) excision or surgical removal
- D) a and c

Chapter 12-Urinary System

Using the list of terms below, create flash cards to learn the meaning of each prefix, prior to completing the assessment that follows.

a-	Necr/o
Albumin/o	Nephr/o
an-	Noct/i
Angi/o	Olig/o
anti-	-oma
Arteri/o	-ostomy
Azot/o	Peri-
Bacteri/o	-plasty
Cali/o	-poiesis
Calic/o	Poly-
Cyst/o	-ptosis
dia-	Py/o
-dilation	Pyel/o
Dips/o	Ren/o
dys-	retro-
En-	-rrhea
-esis	-scelerosis
Glomerul/o	-spasm
Glyc/o	-stenosis
Glycos/o	Tom/o
Hydr/o	-tomy
-ia	Tox/o
Isch/o	Trigon/o
Ket/o	-tripsy
Keton/o	-trophy
Lith/o	Ur/o
-lithiasis	Ureter/o
-lithotomy	Urethr/o
-lysis	-uria
Meat/o	Urin/o
-megaly	Vesic/o

Multiple Choice

Circle the most appropriate response.

____ 1. **The combining form that means kidney is**
   A) nephr/o
   B) vesic/o
   C) ren/o
   D) a and c

____ 2. **The combining form pyel/o is defined as**
   A) bladder
   B) renal pelvis
   C) urethral meatus
   D) ureter

____ 3. **The combining form that means sugar is**
   A) hidr/o
   B) hydr/o
   C) glyc/o
   D) a and c

____ 4. **The combining form that means urea, nitrogen is**
   A) olig/o
   B) urin/o
   C) son/o
   D) azot/o

____ 5. **The combining form that means stone, calculus is**
   A) blast/o
   B) lith/o
   C) tom/o
   D) azot/o

____ 6. **The combining form that means water is**
   A) glyc/o
   B) hidr/o
   C) hydr/o
   D) hem/o

_____ 7. **The combining form cyst/o means**
   A) cell
   B) urinary bladder
   C) to secrete
   D) female

_____ 8. **The combining form ur/o means**
   A) urine
   B) uroma
   C) water
   D) fluid

_____ 9. **The combining form angi/o is**
   A) vessel
   B) duct
   C) vein
   D) either a or b

_____ 10. **The combining form that means artery is**
   A) arti/o
   B) aort/o
   C) angi/o
   D) arteri/o

_____ 11. **The combining form that means death is**
   A) necr/o
   B) pachy/o
   C) coni/o
   D) aut/o

_____ 12. **The combining form that means urethra is**
   A) uretr/o
   B) urethr/o
   C) uter/o
   D) all of the above

_____ 13. **The combining form that means poison is**
   A) tox/o
   B) poison/o
   C) top/o
   D) thyr/o

____ **14. The combining form isch/o means to**
A) yellowish, fatty plaque
B) sound
C) to hold back; back
D) clot

____ **15. The combining form dips/o means**
A) double
B) poison
C) thirst
D) height

____ **16. The prefix peri- means**
A) surrounding
B) half
C) behind
D) inside

____ **17. The prefix poly- is defined as**
A) many
B) without
C) through
D) few

____ **18. The prefix that means without or absence of is**
A) a, an-
B) endo-
C) intra-
D) eu-

____ **19. The prefix that means through, complete is**
A) dia-
B) hyper-
C) dys-
D) pro-

____ **20. The prefix retro- means**
A) back
B) backward
C) behind
D) all of the above

____ 21. The prefix dys- means
   A) bad, painful
   B) difficult, abnormal
   C) a and b
   D) none of the above

____ 22. The prefix that means against is
   A) ante-
   B) anti-
   C) auto-
   D) cata-

____ 23. The suffix that means blood condition is
   A) -ectomy
   B) -oma
   C) -emia
   D) none of the above

____ 24. The suffix that means repair is
   A) -angio
   B) -plasty
   C) -tomy
   D) all of the above

____ 25. The suffix that means hardening is
   A) -malacia
   B) -sclerosis
   C) -penia
   D) -crit

____ 26. The suffix -ptosis means
   A) drooping
   B) sagging
   C) proplase
   D) all of the above

____ 27. The suffix that means nourishment, development is
   A) -esis
   B) -megaly
   C) -trophy
   D) -iasis

_____ **28. The suffix that means cutting into is**
A) -ostomy
B) -tomy
C) a and b
D) none of the above

_____ **29. The suffix -lysis means**
A) breakdown
B) destruction
C) separation
D) all of the above

_____ **30. The suffix that means little, small is**
A) -ole
B) -ule
C) -ia
D) a and b only

_____ **31. The suffix -megaly means**
A) small
B) enlarged
C) a and b
D) none of the above

_____ **32. The suffix that means to flow, discharge is**
A) -menes
B) -rrhapy
C) -rrhea
D) -rrhexis

_____ **33. The suffix that means suturing, repairing is**
A) -megaly
B) -trophy
C) -rrhaphy
D) -esis

_____ **34. The suffix -dilation means to**
A) widening
B) stretching
C) expanding
D) all of the above

____ **35. The suffix that means sudden, involuntary contraction of muscles is**

    A) -stasis
    B) -spasm
    C) -ptosis
    D) -lysis

____ **36. The suffix -stenosis means**

    A) tightening
    B) stricture
    C) narrowing
    D) all of the above

____ **37. The suffix that means new opening**

    A) -ectomy
    B) -ostomy
    C) -tomy
    D) -sthenia

____ **38. The prefix en- means**

    A) in
    B) within
    C) out
    D) a and b

____ **39. The suffix -lithiasis means**

    A) condition of stones
    B) stones
    C) condition
    D) none of the above

____ **40. The suffix -lithotomy means**

    A) incision into a bone
    B) excision of a stone
    C) incision for removal of a stone
    D) none of the above

____ **41. The suffix that means the substance that forms is**

    A) -poiesis
    B) -poietin
    C) -poikil/o
    D) -pod/o

____ 42. The suffix that means to crush is
A) -tripsy
B) -crush
C) -trip
D) none of the above

____ 43. The suffix that means the urination; condition of urine
A) -urope
B) -uria
C) -urine
D) -urination

____ 44. The combining form that means calix (calyx)
A) cali/o
B) calic/o
C) a and b
D) none of the above

____ 45. The combining form that means glomerulus
A) cyst/o
B) glomerul/o
C) meat/o
D) capn/o

____ 46. The combining form meat/o means
A) meatus
B) meat
C) stenosis
D) none of the above

____ 47. The combining form that means trigone (region of the bladder)
A) region/o
B) cyt/o
C) cyst/o
D) trigon/o

____ 48. The combining form that means ureter is
A) ureter/o
B) urethr/o
C) vesic/o
D) ur/o

____ **49. The combining form that means urinary bladder is**
A) vesic/o
B) cyt/o
C) ren/o
D) ureter/o

____ **50. The combining form that means ketone bodies is**
A) ket/o
B) keton/o
C) jeton/e
D) a and b

____ **51. The combining form that means bacteria is**
A) ur/o
B) bacteri/o
C) bacteri/a
D) none of the above

____ **52. The combining form that means night is**
A) noct/i
B) night/o
C) sleep/o
D) all of the above

____ **53. The combining form that means scanty is**
A) azot/o
B) dips/o
C) py/o
D) olig/o

____ **54. The combining form that means pus is**
A) pus/o
B) pus/i
C) py/o
D) pyo/o

___ 55. The combining form that means urine is
A) up/o
B) urin/o
C) urine/o
D) urea/o

___ 56. The combining form albumin/o means
A) albumin
B) fat
C) starch
D) sugar

___ 57. The combining form that means glucose;sugar is
A) glycos/o
B) gnos/o
C) gloss/o
D) all of the above

___ 58. The combining form that means to cut is
A) incis/o
B) ot/o
C) ect/o
D) tom/o

Chapter 13-Reproductive System

Using the list of terms below, create flash cards to learn the meaning of each prefix, prior to completing the assessment that follows.

Amni/o	Intra-	-plasia
Andr/o	-itis	Primi-
Ante-	Lact/o	Prostat/o
-arche	-lysis	Pseudo-
Balan/o	-lytic	-ptosis
Bi-	mamm/o	Py/o
-cele	Mast/o	Retro-
Cephal/o	Men/o	-rraphy
Cervic/o	Metr/o	-rrhea
Chori/o	Metri/o	Salping/o
Chorion/o	Multi-	-salpinx
Colp/o	My/o	Semin/i
Cry/o	Myom/o	Sperm/o
Crypt/o	Nat/I	Spermata/o
Culd/o	Nulli-	-stenosis
Dys-	Olig/o	Terat/o
-ectasis	-one	Test/o
-ectomy	Oophor/o	-tocia
Endo-	Orch/o	-tomy
Epididym/o	Orchid/o	-tresia
Episi/o	-ostomy	-trophy
Galact/o	Ov/o	Uni-
-gen	Ovari/o	Ureter/o
-genesis	Ovul/o	Uter/o
-genic	Oxy-	Vagin/o
Gon/o	-pareunia	Varic/o
-gravida	-parous	Vas/o
Gynec/o	-pepsi	-version
Hydr/o	Peri-	Vulv/o
Hyster/o	Perine/o	Zo/o
In-	Phor/o	

Multiple Choice

Circle the most appropriate response.

____ 1. **The prefix that means many is**
A) nulli-
B) multi-
C) many-
D) all of the above

____ 2. **The prefix that means one is**
A) bi-
B) uni-
C) tri-
D) tetra-

____ 3. **The prefix that means surrounding, around**
A) endo-
B) pro-
C) peri-
D) hypo-

____ 4. **The prefix nulli- means**
A) first
B) one
C) none
D) nulli

____ 5. **The prefix oxy- means**
A) swift
B) sharp
C) acid
D) all of the above

____ 6. **The prefix primi- means**
A) primitive
B) first
C) last
D) second

___ 7. **The prefix that means into, not is**
   A) endo-
   B) in-
   C) bi-
   D) indo-

___ 8. **The prefix that means false**
   A) pseudo-
   B) re-
   C) retro-
   D) sub-

___ 9. **The prefix that means in; within**
   A) uni-
   B) retro-
   C) ante-
   D) endo-

___ 10. **The prefix retro- means**
   A) back
   B) backward
   C) behind
   D) all of the above

___ 11. **The prefix intra- means**
   A) between
   B) into
   C) within
   D) b and c

___ 12. **The prefix that means two**
   A) bio-
   B) bi-
   C) lateral-
   D) tri-

___ 13. **The prefix dys- means**
   A) bad, painful
   B) difficult, abnormal
   C) a and b
   D) none of the above

____ **14. The prefix ante- means**
A) against
B) after
C) before
D) without

____ **15. The suffix that means incision, to cut into is**
A) -ostomy
B) -tomy
C) a and b
D) none of the above

____ **16. The suffix that means repair is**
A) -angio
B) -plasty
C) -tomy
D) all of the above

____ **17. The suffix that means to flow, discharge is**
A) -menes
B) -rrhapy
C) -rrhea
D) -rrhexis

____ **18. The suffix -tresia means**
A) to turn
B) bursting forth
C) begining
D) opening

____ **19. The suffix that means to bear; bring forth**
A) -gravida
B) -parous
C) -pareunia
D) -plasia

____ **20. The suffix -arche means**
A) end
B) before
C) middle
D) beginning

____ **21. The suffix -gravida means**
A) sexual intercourse
B) pregnant woman
C) opening
D) bursting forth

____ **22. The suffix that means inflammation is**
A) -ion
B) -ist
C) -itis
D) -logy

____ **23. The suffix -ectomy is defined as**
A) surgical repair
B) instrument used to cut
C) excision or surgical removal
D) a and c

____ **24. The suffix that means stretching; dilation; expansion is**
A) -ectasis
B) -centesis
C) -capnia
D) -pnea

____ **25. The suffix that means fallopian tube**
A) -plasy
B) -stenosis
C) -tomy
D) -salpinx

____ **26. The suffix -tocia is defined as**
A) birth
B) before
C) labor
D) either a or c

____ **27. The suffix -ptosis means**
A) drooping
B) sagging
C) proplase
D) all of the above

____ **28. The suffix -pareunia means**
A) orgasm
B) sexual intercourse
C) opening
D) to turn

____ **29. The suffix -plasia is defined as**
A) formation, development, growth
B) causing
C) static
D) abnormal condition

____ **30. The suffix for producing; forming is**
A) -genesis
B) -ous
C) -grape
D) -oid

____ **31. The suffix -version means**
A) present
B) past
C) to turn
D) edition

____ **32. The suffix -stenosis means**
A) tightening
B) stricture
C) narrowing
D) all of the above

____ **33. The suffix that means hernia is**
A) -cyte
B) -cele
C) -centesis
D) -coccus

____ **34. The combining form myom/o means**
A) muscle tumor
B) midwife
C) ovary
D) egg

____ **35. The combining form that means uterus is**
   A)   urethr/o
   B)   ureter/o
   C)   uter/o
   D)   all of the above

____ **36. The combining form men/o means**
   A)   last, ending
   B)   menstruation
   C)   first, beginning
   D)   regular

____ **37. The combining form that means uterus is**
   A)   hyster/o
   B)   ureter/o
   C)   vulvo
   D)   a and b

____ **38. The combining form that means pus**
   A)   pus/o
   B)   pus/i
   C)   py/o
   D)   pyo/o

____ **39. The combining form perine/o means**
   A)   uterus
   B)   ovary
   C)   pregnant
   D)   perineum

____ **40. The combining form chori/o means**
   A)   color
   B)   green
   C)   chorion
   D)   choirion

____ **41. The combining form that means woman is**
   A)   andr/o
   B)   uter/o
   C)   gynec/o
   D)   a and c

____ **42. The combining form that means egg is**

A) ov/o
B) ovari/o
C) ovul/o
D) a and c

____ **43. The combining form that means vulva is**

A) valv/o
B) vulv/o
C) vilv/o
D) velv/o

____ **44. The combining form culd/o means**

A) culdom
B) cul-de-sac
C) vulva
D) uterus

____ **45. The combining form nat/i means**

A) navel
B) pregnancy
C) embryo
D) birth

____ **46. The combining form that means milk is**

A) milk/o
B) galact/o
C) lact/o
D) b and c

____ **47. The combining form that means uterus is**

A) metr/o
B) metri/o
C) my/o
D) a and b

____ **48. The combining form that means scanty is**

A) olig/o
B) ov/o
C) man/o
D) scant/o

____ 49. The combining form that means egg is
- A) perine/o
- B) o/o
- C) ovari/o
- D) ovul/o

____ 50. The combining form colp/o means
- A) vagina
- B) uterus
- C) ovary
- D) cul-de-sac

____ 51. The combining form that means head is
- A) encephal/o
- B) cephal/o
- C) enter/o
- D) cerebr/o

____ 52. The combining form that means muscle
- A) mamm/o
- B) muc/o
- C) morph/o
- D) my/o

____ 53. The combining form that means neck; cervix (neck of uterus)
- A) neck/o
- B) cervic/o
- C) chrom/o
- D) coccyg/o

____ 54. The combining form phor/o means
- A) to carry
- B) to bear
- C) to give
- D) to take

____ 55. The combining form that means breast is
- A) metr/o
- B) mast/o
- C) mamm/o
- D) b and c

____ **56. The combining form that means midwife is**
    A) nat/i
    B) obstetr/o
    C) olig/o
    D) ov/o

____ **57. The combining form episi/o means**
    A) milk
    B) uterus
    C) cul-de-sac
    D) vulva

____ **58. The combining form that means ovary is**
    A) oophor/o
    B) episi/o
    C) colp/o
    D) culd/o

____ **59. The combining form that means the sac surrounding the embryo in the uterus is**
    A) agor/a
    B) amni/o
    C) angi/o
    D) aden/o

____ **60. The combining form salping/o means**
    A) cervix
    B) auditory (eustachian tube)
    C) fallopian tube
    D) b and c

____ **61. The combining form chorion/o means**
    A) fetus
    B) sac
    C) fluid
    D) chorion

____ **62. The combining form that means vagina is**
    A) valv/o
    B) uter/o
    C) gynec/o
    D) vagin/o

____ **63. The suffix means urinary bladder; sac of fluid**
  A) -plasty
  B) -sac
  C) -cyesis
  D) none of the above

____ **64. The suffix that means to suture is**
  A) -sew
  B) -suture
  C) -rraphy
  D) all of the above

____ **65. The combining form that means ovary is**
  A) ov/o
  B) ovari/o
  C) o/o
  D) all of the above

____ **66. The suffix that means incision, to cut into is**
  A) -ostomy
  B) -tomy
  C) a and b
  D) none of the above

____ **67. The suffix that means to flow, discharge is**
  A) -menes
  B) -rrhapy
  C) -rrhea
  D) -rrhexis

____ **68. The suffix that means hormone is**
  A) -one
  B) -hormone
  C) -oid
  D) -optic

____ **69. The suffix that means fixation is**
  A) -pepsi
  B) -pexy
  C) -spexy
  D) -fixation

___ **70. The suffix that means to reduce, destroy**
A) -lytico
B) -lytic
C) -lobular
D) none of the above

___ **71. The suffix -genic means**
A) pertaining to
B) genetics
C) produced by
D) a and c

___ **72. The suffix that means to create an artificial opening**
A) -ectomy
B) -ostomy
C) -tomy
D) -sthenia

___ **73. The suffix that means nourishment, development is**
A) -esis
B) -megaly
C) -trophy
D) -iasis

___ **74. The suffix -ectomy is defined as**
A) surgical repair
B) instrument used to cut
C) excision or surgical removal
D) a and c

___ **75. The suffix -lysis means**
A) breakdown
B) destruction
C) separation
D) all of the above

___ **76. The suffix -gen means**
A) grow
B) formlin
C) produced by or in
D) b and c

___ 77. The suffix -plasia is defined as
A) formation, development, growth
B) causing
C) static
D) abnormal condition

___ 78. The suffix for producing; forming is
A) -genesis
B) -ous
C) -grape
D) -oid

___ 79. The suffix that means hernia is
A) -cyte
B) -cele
C) -centesis
D) -coccus

___ 80. The combining form that means male is
A) sperm/o
B) test/o
C) vas/o
D) andr/o

___ 81. The combining form that means water is
A) glyc/o
B) urin/o
C) hydr/o
D) hem/o

___ 82. The combining form that means testis is
A) orch/o
B) orchid/o
C) a and b only
D) none of the above

___ 83. The combining form that means vessel or duct is
A) vas/o
B) orchid/o
C) balan/o
D) vesicul/o

____ **84. The combining form that means hidden is**
A) coni/o
B) rhytid/o
C) xer/o
D) crypt/o

____ **85. The combining form that means spermatoza; semen**
A) sperm/o
B) spermat/o
C) spermata/o
D) a and b

____ **86. The combining form gon/o means**
A) gonus
B) gone
C) gono
D) seed

____ **87. The combining form that means semen; seed**
A) semin/i
B) test/o
C) seed/o
D) a and c

____ **88. The combining form that means glans penis is**
A) vesicul/o
B) prostat/o
C) balan/o
D) vas/o

____ **89. The combining form terat/o means**
A) animal
B) monster
C) vessel
D) four

____ **90. The combining form that means testis is**
A) balan/o
B) vesicul/o
C) prostat/o
D) test/o

____ **91. The combining form that mean cold is**
A) balan/o
B) cry/o
C) crypt/o
D) gon/o

____ **92. The combining form epididym/o means**
A) epidid
B) epidymis
C) epididymis
D) all of the above

____ **93. The combining for that means animal life is**
A) animal/o
B) zo/o
C) a and b
D) none of the above

____ **94. The combining form that means varicose veins**
A) vas/o
B) varicu/o
C) varic/o
D) all of the above

____ **95. The combining form that means prostate gland is**
A) balan/o
B) prostat/o
C) prostrat/o
D) vas/o

Chapter 14-Endocrine System

Using the list of terms below, create flash cards to learn the meaning of each prefix, prior to completing the assessment that follows.

Aden/o	Myx/o
Adren/o	Natr/o
Adrenal/o	-oid
-agon	-osis
Andr/o	Oxy-
Calc/o	Pan-
Cortic/o	Pancreat/o
Crin/o	Panreact/o
Dips/o	parthyroid/o
-ectomy	Phys/o
-emia	-physis
Estr/o	Pituitary/o
Eu-	Poly-
-genic	-stasis
Gluc/o	Ster/o
Glyc/o	Stomat/o
Gonad/o	Tetra-
Home/o	Thyr/o
Hormon/o	Thyroid/o
Hyper-	Toc/o
Hypo-	-tocin
-in	Toxic/o
-ine	Tri-
Kal/i	-tropin
Lact/o	Ur/o
-megaly	-uria

Multiple Choice

Circle the most appropriate response.

_____ 1. **The prefix that means excessive**
   A) hypo-
   B) hyper-
   C) sub-
   D) trans-

_____ 2. **The prefix that means deficient; below; under**
   A) trans-
   B) hyper-
   C) hypo-
   D) pro-

_____ 3. **The suffix -genic means**
   A) pertaining to
   B) genetics
   C) produced by or in
   D) a and c

_____ 4. **The suffix -ectomy is defined as**
   A) surgical repair
   B) instrument used to cut
   C) excision or surgical removal
   D) a and c

_____ 5. **The suffix that means blood condition is**
   A) -ectomy
   B) -oma
   C) -emia
   D) none of the above

_____ 6. **The suffix that means condition is**
   A) -itis
   B) -osis
   C) -pathy
   D) -emia

____ 7. **The suffix that means control, stop, place is**
   A) -osis
   B) -plasm
   C) -genesis
   D) -stasis

____ 8. **The suffix that means resembling is**
   A) -ose
   B) -ous
   C) -oid
   D) -tic

____ 9. **The suffix -megaly means**
   A) small
   B) enlarged
   C) a and b
   D) none of the above

____ 10. **The prefix poly- is defined as**
   A) many, much
   B) without
   C) through
   D) few

____ 11. **The prefix that means all**
   A) peri-
   B) pan-
   C) per-
   D) para-

____ 12. **The suffix that means to grow**
   A) -growth
   B) -physis
   C) -grew
   D) none of the above

____ 13. **The suffix that means the urination; condition of urine**
   A) -urope
   B) -uria
   C) -urine
   D) -urination

____ **14. The suffix -in,-ine means**
A) endocrine
B) secrete
C) a substance
D) all of the above

____ **15. The prefix that means four**
A) trio-
B) tri-
C) tetra-
D) all of the above

____ **16. The prefix that means three**
A) tri-
B) quadri-
C) tetra-
D) bi-

____ **17. The prefix that means good, normal**
A) normo-
B) eu-
C) ex-
D) brady-

____ **18. The suffix that means to assemble is**
A) -ectomy
B) -megaly
C) -agon
D) -assembl

____ **19. The suffix that means labor; birth is**
A) -pseudo
B) -tocin
C) -uria
D) all of the above

____ **20. The suffix that means to stimulate; act on is**
A) -megaly
B) -agon
C) -emia
D) -tropin

____ **21. The combining form cortic/o means**
- A) calcium
- B) cortisol
- C) cortex
- D) endocrine

____ **22. The combining form thyr/o means**
- A) parathyroid gland
- B) thyroid gland
- C) endocrine gland
- D) cortex

____ **23. The combining form dips/o means**
- A) double
- B) poison
- C) thirst
- D) height

____ **24. The combining form that means poison is**
- A) kal/i
- B) acr/o
- C) toxic/o
- D) calc/i

____ **25. The combining form that means calcium is**
- A) kal/i
- B) natr/o
- C) dips/o
- D) calc/o

____ **26. The combining form that means male is**
- A) sperm/o
- B) test/o
- C) vas/o
- D) andr/o

____ **27. The combining form aden/o means**
- A) wrinkles
- B) life
- C) gland
- D) scaly

_____ **28. The combining form ur/o means**
A) urine
B) urinary tract
C) water
D) a and b

_____ **29. The combining form crin/o means**
A) endocrine gland
B) exocrine gland
C) secrete
D) adrenal glad

_____ **30. The combining form that means sugar is**
A) hidr/o
B) hydr/o
C) glyc/o
D) a and c

_____ **31. The combining form that means adrenal gland is**
A) adren/o
B) adrenal/o
C) a and b
D) aden/o

_____ **32. The combining form that means female is**
A) andr/o
B) home/o
C) estr/o
D) all of the above

_____ **33. The combining form that means sugar is**
A) gulc/o
B) glug/o
C) gluc/o
D) all of the above

_____ **34. The combining form that means sex gland is**
A) kal/i
B) home/o
C) gonad/o
D) lact/o

____ **35. The combining form home/o means**
- A) sameness
- B) unlike
- C) different
- D) all of the above

____ **36. The combining form that means potassium is**
- A) potass/o
- B) kal/i
- C) calc/i
- D) all of the above

____ **37. The combining form that means milk is**
- A) milk/o
- B) lacta/o
- C) lcat/o
- D) lact/o

____ **38. The combining form myx/o means**
- A) milk
- B) pus
- C) mucus
- D) body

____ **39. The combining form natr/o means**
- A) sugar
- B) salt
- C) potassium
- D) sodium

____ **40. The combining form that means pancreas is**
- A) pancreat/o
- B) somat/o
- C) ster/o
- D) none of the above

____ **41. The combining form parthyroid/o means**
- A) gland
- B) thyroid
- C) parathyroid glands
- D) none of the above

____ **42. The combining form pituitar/o means**
A) pituitary gland
B) gland
C) pituitary
D) none of the above

____ **43. The combining form that means body is**
A) stomat/o
B) somat/o
C) bod/o
D) all of the above

____ **44. The combining form that means solid structure is**
A) ster/o
B) toc/o
C) thyr/o
D) lact/o

____ **45. The combining form that means thyroid gland is**
A) thyroid/o
B) aden/o
C) ster/o
D) toc/o

____ **46. The combining form toc/o means**
A) labor
B) birth
C) place
D) a and b

____ **47. The prefix that means swift;sharp;acid**
A) oxy-
B) oxysm-
C) ox-
D) all of the above

____ **48. The combining form that means hormone is**
A) hurmon/o
B) hurmone/o
C) hormon/o
D) none of the above

____ **49. The combining form that means pancreatic hormone is**
    A) insulin/o
    B) hormon/o
    C) panreact/o
    D) none of the above

____ **50. The combining form that means growing is**
    A) phys/o
    B) stern/o
    C) gluc/o
    D) dips/o

Chapter 15-Nervous System

Using the list of terms below, create flash cards to learn the meaning of each prefix, prior to completing the assessment that follows.

A, An-	Hyper-	-phagia
-algesia	Hypo-	-phasia
-algia	-in	-plegia
Angi/o	-ine	Polio-
-blast	Intra-	Poly-
Caus/o	-it is	Pont/o
-cele	Kines/o	-praxia
Cephal/o	Kinesi/o	-ptosis
Cerebell/o	-kinesia	Quadri-
Cerebr/o	-kinesis	Radicul/o
Comat/o	-lepsy	-sclerosis
Crani/o	Lept/o	Spin/o
Cry/o	Lex/o	-sthenia
Dur/o	Mening/o	Sub-
Dys-	Meningi/o	Syncop/o
Encephal/o	Micro-	Tax/o
Epi-	My/o	Thalam/o
Esthesi/o	Myel/o	Thec/o
-esthesia	Narc/o	-tomy
Gli/o	Neur/o	Troph/o
-grahpy	-ose	-trophy
-gram	Para-	Vag/o
Hemi-	-paresis	
Hydr/o	-pathy	

Multiple Choice

Circle the most appropriate response.

_____ 1. **The combining form narc/o means**
   A) numbness
   B) stupor
   C) sleep
   D) all of the above

_____ 2. **The suffix -plegia is defined as**
   A) vision
   B) paralysis
   C) abnormal fear or aversion
   D) pressure

_____ 3. **The suffix that means speech is**
   A) -phasia
   B) -pexy
   C) -capnia
   D) -eal

_____ 4. **The suffix that means movement is**
   A) -kinesia
   B) -kinesis
   C) -kinder
   D) a and b

_____ 5. **The suffix that means -lepsy means**
   A) eplilepsy
   B) seizure
   C) seixzure
   D) all of the above

_____ 6. **The suffix -ptosis means**
   A) drooping
   B) sagging
   C) proplase
   D) all of the above

____ 7. **The combining form gli/o means**
   A) glius
   B) glue
   C) gyrus
   D) none of the above

____ 8. **The prefix micro- means**
   A) large
   B) enlarged
   C) small
   D) all of the above

____ 9. **The combining form that means nervous sensation**
   A) esthesi/o
   B) end/o
   C) estr/o
   D) a and b

____ 10. **The combining form lex/o means**
   A) slender
   B) phrase
   C) word
   D) b and c

____ 11. **The sufix -gram means**
   A) process of recording
   B) record
   C) a and b
   D) none of the above

____ 12. **The suffix -paresis is defined as**
   A) slight paralysis
   B) sensitivity
   C) seizure
   D) softening

____ 13. **The combining form that means dura mater is**
   A) duro/o
   B) dur/a
   C) dur/o

D) all of the above

____ 14. The suffix -algesia means
A) difficult
B) painful
C) pain
D) sensitivity to pain

____ 15. The combining form cerebr/o means
A) cerebrum
B) head
C) skull
D) cerebullum

____ 16. The combining form spin/o is defined as
A) spine
B) backbone
C) flesh
D) a and b

____ 17. The combining form that means water is
A) glyc/o
B) urin/o
C) hydr/o
D) hem/o

____ 18. The combining form that means to cut off, cut short is
A) spin/o
B) syncop/o
C) syncopo
D) syncope

____ 19. The combining form that means thalamus is
A) thalam/o
B) thlaam/o
C) thalam/a
D) all of the above

____ 20. The combining form lept/o means
A) smoth
B) to seizure
C) seizure

D) thin, slender

____ 21. The suffix that means pain is
A) -cele
B) -pexy
C) -spasm
D) -algia

____ 22. The prefix that means gray matter (of brain or spinal cord) is
A) poli-
B) my-
C) poly-
D) polio-

____ 23. The suffix -in,-ine means
A) endocrine
B) secrete
C) a substance
D) all of the above

____ 24. The combining form tax/o means
A) order
B) coordination
C) taxi
D) a and b

____ 25. The combining form that means cold is
A) balan/o
B) cry/o
C) crypt/o
D) gon/o

____ 26. The suffix -esthesia is defined as a
A) break
B) split, fissure
C) nervous sensation
D) growth

____ 27. The prefix that means deficient; below; under
A) trans-
B) hyper-
C) hypo-

D) pro-

28. The suffix that means hardening is
A) -malacia
B) -sclerosis
C) -penia
D) -crit

29. The suffix that means tumor is
A) -opsy
B) -oma
C) -cyte
D) -al

30. The prefix poly- is defined as
A) many
B) without
C) through
D) few

31. The combining form that means sensitivty to pain is
A) -algesia
B) alges/o
C) caus/o
D) none of the above

32. The suffix that means inflammation is
A) -ion
B) -ist
C) -itis
D) -logy

33. The suffix -phagia is defined as
A) surgical repair
B) softening
C) disease or abnormal state
D) eating or swallowing

34. The combining form radicul/o means
A) nerve root
B) back
C) pain

D) all of the above

___ 35. The combining form troph/o means
A) nourishment
B) development
C) a and b
D) none of the above

___ 36. The suffix -ose means
A) pertaining to
B) full of
C) a and b
D) none of the above

___ 37. The combining form that means nerve is
A) hepat/o
B) neur/o
C) gastr/o
D) none of the above

___ 38. The combining form esthesi/o is defined as
A) pain
B) painful
C) difficult
D) nervous sensation

___ 39. The combining form for bone marrow or spinal cord is
A) myel/o
B) myc/o
C) myos/o
D) none of the above

___ 40. The combining form angi/o means
A) vessel
B) ductus
C) vein
D) either a or b

___ 41. The suffix that means hernia
A) -cyte
B) -cele
C) -centesis

D) -coccus

____ 42. The combining form that means brain is
A) cephal/o
B) encephal/o
C) psych/o
D) a and c

____ 43. The combining form that means head is
A) encephal/o
B) cephal/o
C) enter/o
D) cerebr/o

____ 44. The prefix hemi- is defined as
A) four
B) half
C) before
D) two

____ 45. The combining form cerebell/o means
A) cerebrum
B) cerebellum
C) a and b
D) none of the above

____ 46. The suffix that means the process of recording
A) -gram
B) -graph
C) -grahpy
D) -all of the above

____ 47. The suffix that means the process of cutting
A) -ostomy
B) -tomy
C) -ology
D) -scopy

____ 48. The combining form that means muscle is
A) mamm/o
B) muc/o
C) morph/o

D) my/o

____ **49. The combining form that means movement, motion is**
A) kines/o
B) kinesi/o
C) ankyl/o
D) a and b

____ **50. The suffix that means disease**
A) -ology
B) -pathy
C) -tomy
D) -ion

____ **51. The combining form that means vagus nerve is**
A) valv/o
B) ven/o
C) vag/o
D) vaso

____ **52. The suffix -praxia means**
A) paxil
B) praxial
C) action
D) strength

____ **53. The prefix that means near; beside**
A) neo-
B) para-
C) per-
D) meta-

____ **54. The prefix that means without or absence of is**
A) a, an-
B) endo-
C) intra-
D) eu-

____ **55. The suffix -sthenia is defined as a**

A) break
B) split, fissure

    C) strength
    D) growth

____ **56. The combining form that means burn or burning is**
    A) burn/o
    B) caus/o
    C) comat/o
    D) dur/o

____ **57. The prefix that means four is**
    A) bi-
    B) tri-
    C) uni-
    D) quadri-

____ **58. The combining form that means sheath is**
    A) vag/o
    B) tax/o
    C) troph/o
    D) thec/o

____ **59. The prefix that means below,under is**
    A) sub-
    B) trans-
    C) re-
    D) peri-

____ **60. The prefix dys- means**
    A) bad, painful
    B) difficult, abnormal
    C) a and b
    D) none of the above

____ **61. The suffix -blast means**
    A) to blow up
    B) embryonic
    C) immature
    D) b and c only

____ **62. The combining form pont/o means**
    A) pons
    B) pontine
    C) pono

D) all of the above

____ **63. The prefix that means on, upon, over is**
A) intra-
B) pro-
C) epi-
D) sub-

____ **64. The combining form that means meninges is**
A) mening/o
B) meningi/o
C) meng/o
D) a and b

____ **65. The prefix that means above; excessive**
A) hypo-
B) hyper-
C) sub-
D) trans-

____ **66. The prefix intra- means**
A) between
B) into
C) within
D) b and c

____ **67. The combining form that means glue is**
A) gastr/o
B) gli/o
C) glue/o
D) all of the above

____ **68. The suffix that means nourishment, development is**
A) -esis
B) -megaly
C) -trophy
D) -iasis

____ **69. The combining form that means deep sleep is**
A) somn/o
B) sleep/o
C) comat/o

D) all of the above

____ 70. The combining form that means skull is
A) encephal/o
B) cephal/o
C) skull/o
D) crani/o

Chapter 16-Eye & Ear

Using the list of terms below, create flash cards to learn the meaning of each prefix, prior to completing the assessment that follows.

Acous/o	nyct/o
-acusis	Ocul/o
Ambly/o	Ophthalm/o
Anis/o	-opia
Aque/o	-opsia
Audi/o	opt/o
Audit/o	optic/o
Aur/o	Ossicul/o
Auricul/o	Ot/o
Blephar/o	-otia
Cochle/o	Papill/o
Conjunctiv/o	Phac/o
Cor/o	Phak/o
Corne/o	-phobia
-cusis	Phot/o
Cycl/o	-plegic
Dacry/o	Presby/o
Dipil/o	Pupil/o
Glauc/o	Retin/o
Ir/o	Salping/o
Irid/o	Scler/o
Kerat/o	Scot/o
Lacrim/o	Staped/o
Light/o	-tropia
mastoid/o	Tympan/o
Mi/o	Uve/o
Myc/o	Vestibul/o
Mydr/o	Vitre/o
Myring/o	Xer/o

Multiple Choice

Circle the most appropriate response.

_____ 1. **The suffix that means hearing is**
    A) -acusis
    B) -opia
    C) -cusis
    D) a and c

_____ 2. **The suffix that means vision is**
    A) -opia
    B) -cusis
    C) -opsia
    D) a and c

_____ 3. **The suffix -otia means**
    A) ear
    B) condition
    C) ear condition
    D) inflammation

_____ 4. **The that means to turn is**
    A) -turna
    B) -trophy
    C) -tropia
    D) -plegic

_____ 5. **The suffix that means fear is**
    A) -plegia
    B) -phobia
    C) -tropia
    D) -otia

_____ 6. **The suffix that means paralysis; palsy**
    A) -phobia
    B) -cusis
    C) -opia
    D) -plegic

_____ 7. **The combining form ophthalm/o means**
   A) lens
   B) vision
   C) eyelid
   D) eye

_____ 8. **The combining form myc/o means**
   A) fungus
   B) muscle
   C) oil
   D) dust

_____ 9. **The combining form kerat/o means**
   A) skin
   B) horny
   C) hard
   D) b and c

_____ 10. **The combining form that means dry is**
   A) hidr/o
   B) xer/o
   C) coni/o
   D) all of the above

_____ 11. **The combining form that means eyelid is**
   A) blephar/o
   B) kerat/o
   C) opt/o
   D) cor/o

_____ 12. **The combining form that means cornea is**
   A) kerat/o
   B) corne/o
   C) core
   D) a and b

_____ 13. **The combining forms ir/o and irid/o mean**
   A) pupil
   B) iris
   C) eye
   D) retina

_____ 14. **The combining form that means tear or tear duct is**
   A) conjunctiv/o
   B) lacrim/o

C) dacry/o
D) b and c

___ 15. A combining form that means double is
   A) bin/o
   B) dipl/o
   C) opia
   D) cry/o

___ 16. The combining form acous/o means
   A) balance
   B) ear
   C) hearing
   D) a and b

___ 17. The combining form that means eardrum is
   A) audi/o
   B) tympan/o
   C) ot/o
   D) aur/i

___ 18. The combining form staped/o means
   A) ossicles
   B) mastoid bone
   C) stapes
   D) malleus

___ 19. The combining form that means typanic membrane is
   A) myring/o
   B) aur/o
   C) labyrinth/o
   D) ot/o

___ 20. The combining form ot/o means
   A) ear
   B) eardrum
   C) hearing
   D) middle ear bone

___ 21. The combining form that means hearing is
   A) audi/o
   B) ot/o
   C) audit/o
   D) a and c

____ **22. The combining forms aur/o and auricul/o mean**
    A) ear
    B) hearing
    C) eardrum
    D) none of the above

____ **23. The combining form ocul/o means**
    A) tear
    B) eye
    C) vision
    D) iris

____ **24. The combining form that means dim; dull is**
    A) dim/o
    B) dull/o
    C) ambly/o
    D) all of the above

____ **25. The combining form that means unequal is**
    A) is/o
    B) anis/o
    C) equa/o
    D) all of the above

____ **26. The combining form that means water is**
    A) hidr/o
    B) aque/o
    C) hyp/o
    D) hyper/o

____ **27. The combining form conjunctiv/o means**
    A) ear
    B) eye
    C) inflammation of the eyelid
    D) conjunctiva

____ **28. The combining form that means pupil is**
    A) cor/o
    B) pupil/o
    C) ot/o
    D) blephar/o

____ **29. The combining form cycl/o means**
A) cycle
B) vision
C) ciliary body of the eye
D) a and c

____ **30. The combining form glauc/o**
A) elderly
B) brown
C) gray
D) iris

____ **31. The combining form mastoid/o means**
A) ear
B) prostrate
C) mastoid process
D) mandibule

____ **32. The combining form that means smaller is**
A) macr/o
B) meg/o
C) mi/o
D) my/o

____ **33. The combining form that means wide is**
A) opt/o
B) macr/o
C) mydr/o
D) none of the above

____ **34. The combining form nyct/o means**
A) day
B) night
C) dry
D) yellow

____ **35. The combining form that means eye; vision is**
A) ot/o
B) optic/o
C) opt/o
D) b and c

____ **36. The combining form ossicul/o means**
  A) ear
  B) eye
  C) ossicle
  D) all of the above

____ **37. The combining form that means eyelid is**
  A) palpebr/o
  B) bephar/o
  C) ot/o
  D) all of the above

____ **38. The combining form that means nipple like; optic disc (disk)**
  A) phac/o
  B) phak/o
  C) papill/o
  D) nippl/o

____ **39. The combining form that means lens of the eye is**
  A) phac/o
  B) phak/o
  C) palpebr/o
  D) a and b

____ **40. The combining form that means light**
  A) son/o
  B) phot/o
  C) light/o
  D) all of the above

____ **41. The combining form presby/o means**
  A) light
  B) sound
  C) eye
  D) old age

____ **42. The combining form that means pupil is**
  A) papill/o
  B) pupil/o
  C) caro/o
  D) retin/o

_____ 43. **The combining form that means retina is**
A) scot/o
B) scler/o
C) salping/o
D) retin/o

_____ 44. **The combining form that means sclera is**
A) retin/o
B) scot/o
C) scler/o
D) sceler/o

_____ 45. **The combining form scot/o means**
A) dry
B) red
C) darkness
D) all of the above

_____ 46. **The combining form that means uvea is**
A) uv/o
B) eve/o
C) uve/o
D) all of the above

_____ 47. **The combining form that means vestibule of the inner ear is**
A) ot/o
B) optic/o
C) vestibu/o
D) vestibul/o

_____ 48. **The combining form that means glass is**
A) xer/o
B) xant/o
C) virtre/o
D) vitre/o

_____ 49. **The combining form salping/o means**
A) cervix
B) auditory (eustachian tube)
C) fallopian tube
D) b and c

_____ 50. **The combining form that means inner part of the ear is**
A) tympan/o

B) myring/o
C) cochle/o
D) none of the above

Answer Key
Medical Terminology:
A Review Guide

Chapter 1 Answers

1.	A		25.	B
2.	C		26.	A
3.	A		27.	B
4.	D		28.	A
5.	C		29.	B
6.	A		30.	A
7.	B		31.	A
8.	C		32.	D
9.	C		33.	B
10.	B		34.	A
11.	D		35.	D
12.	D		36.	A
13.	A		37.	B
14.	C		38.	D
15.	B		39.	B
16.	B		40.	B
17.	B		41.	D
18.	D		42.	A
19.	A		43.	D
20.	D		44.	B
21.	B		45.	B
22.	A		46.	C
23.	C		47.	A
24.	B		48.	C

Chapter 2 Answers

1.	C		21.	D
2.	D		22.	D
3.	C		23.	D
4.	C		24.	A
5.	D		25.	C
6.	D		26.	C
7.	A		27.	C
8.	D		28.	B
9.	A		29.	B
10.	B		30.	B
11.	D		31.	C
12.	B		32.	C
13.	B		33.	A
14.	B		34.	B
15.	D		35.	D
16.	D		36.	C
17.	A		37.	C
18.	A		38.	D
19.	A		39.	C
20.	A		40.	C

1.	C		30.	D
2.	D		31.	D
3.	D		32.	B
4.	B		33.	C
5.	C		34.	C
6.	C		35.	B
7.	C		36.	A
8.	B		37.	C
9.	C		38.	A
10.	B		39.	D
11.	C		40.	D
12.	B		41.	D
13.	B		42.	B
14.	B		43.	C
15.	B		44.	B
16.	A		45.	B
17.	B		46.	D
18.	C		47.	C
19.	C		48.	A
20.	B		49.	D
21.	B		50.	D
22.	D		51.	B
23.	B		52.	B
24.	A		53.	A
25.	B		54.	C
26.	D		55.	B
27.	B		56.	B
28.	A		57.	B
29.	B			

Chapter 4 Answers

1.	D		26.	B
2.	C		27.	A
3.	C		28.	B
4.	C		29.	D
5.	C		30.	A
6.	C		31.	D
7.	D		32.	C
8.	A		33.	A
9.	B		34.	D
10.	B		35.	D
11.	B		36.	D
12.	A		37.	B
13.	D		38.	A
14.	D		39.	D
15.	A		40.	B
16.	B		41.	A
17.	A		42.	C
18.	D		43.	D
19.	D		44.	B
20.	D		45.	D
21.	B		46.	D
22.	A		47.	C
23.	B		48.	C
24.	C		49.	B
25.	C			

Chapter 5 Answers

1. D	19. B
2. B	20. C
3. B	21. B
4. D	22. D
5. C	23. C
6. D	24. D
7. C	25. A
8. D	26. A
9. C	27. D
10. D	28. D
11. D	29. D
12. C	30. C
13. A	31. D
14. A	32. D
15. D	33. B
16. D	34. D
17. D	35. B
18. A	36. D

Chapter 6 Answers

1.	A	32.	A	63.	D
2.	C	33.	B	64.	B
3.	D	34.	C	65.	A
4.	A	35.	B	66.	B
5.	D	36.	A	67.	D
6.	B	37.	C	68.	D
7.	D	38.	C	69.	A
8.	C	39.	D	70.	D
9.	A	40.	A	71.	D
10.	C	41.	D	72.	A
11.	D	42.	D	73.	C
12.	D	43.	D	74.	D
13.	D	44.	D	75.	B
14.	B	45.	C	76.	B
15.	D	46.	C	77.	C
16.	A	47.	C	78.	A
17.	B	48.	C	79.	C
18.	A	49.	B	80.	A
19.	B	50.	B	81.	A
20.	A	51.	C	82.	B
21.	D	52.	B	83.	D
22.	C	53.	D	84.	C
23.	A	54.	B	85.	A
24.	D	55.	C	86.	A
25.	C	56.	D	87.	C
26.	A	57.	D	88	B
27.	B	58.	A	89.	D
28.	D	59.	A	90.	A
29.	B	60.	D	91.	C
30.	C	61.	A	92.	D
31.	D	62.	A		

1.	B		33.	D
2.	C		34.	D
3.	B		35.	B
4.	A		36.	D
5.	A		37.	D
6.	C		38.	A
7.	C		39.	D
8.	B		40.	C
9.	B		41.	C
10.	A		42.	C
11.	C		43.	B
12.	B		44.	C
13.	B		45.	B
14.	A		46.	A
15.	D		47.	A
16.	D		48.	D
17.	B		49.	D
18.	B		50.	D
19.	B		51.	B
20.	B		52.	D
21.	B		53.	D
22.	D		54.	D
23.	D		55.	A
24.	B		56.	D
25.	C		57.	B
26.	C		58.	A
27.	C		59.	B
28.	B		60.	A
29.	D		61.	B
30.	A		62.	C
31.	D		63.	C
32.	A		64.	C

Chapter 8 Answers

1.	A		27.	D
2.	C		28.	A
3.	C		29.	B
4.	B		30.	B
5.	C		31.	B
6.	B		32.	D
7.	D		33.	B
8.	C		34.	D
9.	D		35.	B
10.	D		36.	A
11.	D		37.	A
12.	B		38.	D
13.	B		39.	D
14.	A		40.	C
15.	C		41.	B
16.	A		42.	D
17.	C		43.	B
18.	D		44.	C
19.	D		45.	D
20.	D		46.	C
21.	A		47.	D
22.	A		48.	D
23.	C		49.	A
24.	A		50.	D
25.	C		51.	D
26.	D			

Chapter 9 Answers

1.	A		14.	B
2.	B		15.	B
3.	B		16.	D
4.	C		17.	B
5.	D		18.	B
6.	C		19.	B
7.	C		20.	D
8.	C		21.	B
9.	B		22.	D
10.	B		23.	C
11.	D		24.	C
12.	D		25.	C
13.	B			

Chapter 10 Answers

1.	D	24.	B
2.	C	25.	D
3.	A	26.	A
4.	D	27.	D
5.	B	28.	B
6.	A	29.	A
7.	C	30.	B
8.	A	31.	A
9.	B	32.	D
10.	C	33.	D
11.	B	34.	D
12.	C	35.	D
13.	C	36.	D
14.	A	37.	B
15.	B	38.	C
16.	B	39.	A
17.	D	40.	B
18.	C	41.	C
19.	B	42.	A
20.	D	43.	B
21.	B	44.	C
22.	B	45.	D
23.	C	46.	C

Chapter 11 Answers

1.	B	32.	A	63.	B
2.	D	33.	C	64.	C
3.	B	34.	B	65.	A
4.	A	35.	A	66.	B
5.	D	36.	B	67.	B
6.	C	37.	B	68.	B
7.	C	38.	D	69.	D
8.	B	39.	A	70.	D
9.	D	40.	A	71.	D
10.	C	41.	D	72.	A
11.	B	42.	B	73.	C
12.	D	43.	C	74.	D
13.	C	44.	B	75.	B
14.	C	45.	D	76.	A
15.	D	46.	C	77.	B
16.	B	47.	D	78.	B
17.	D	48.	C	79.	D
18.	A	49.	D	80.	C
19.	A	50.	D	81.	D
20.	C	51.	B	82.	C
21.	D	52.	B	83.	D
22.	C	53.	D	84.	D
23.	C	54.	C	85.	B
24.	B	55.	C	86.	A
25.	D	56.	A	87.	A
26.	A	57.	C	88.	C
27.	D	58.	A	89.	D
28.	A	59.	C	90.	C
29.	B	60.	B	91.	A
30.	C	61.	A	92.	C
31.	A	62.	C		

Chapter 12 Answers

1.	D		30.	D
2.	B		31.	B
3.	C		32.	C
4.	D		33.	D
5.	B		34.	C
6.	C		35.	B
7.	B		36.	D
8.	A		37.	B
9.	A		38.	D
10.	D		39.	A
11.	A		40.	C
12.	B		41.	B
13.	A		42.	A
14.	C		43.	B
15.	C		44.	C
16.	A		45.	B
17.	A		46.	A
18.	A		47.	D
19.	A		48.	A
20.	D		49.	A
21.	C		50.	D
22.	B		51.	B
23.	C		52.	A
24.	B		53.	D
25.	B		54.	C
26.	D		55.	B
27.	C		56.	A
28.	B		57.	A
29.	D		58.	D

Chapter 13 Answers

1.	B	33.	B	65.	B
2.	B	34.	A	66.	B
3.	C	35.	C	67.	C
4.	C	36.	B	68.	A
5.	D	37.	D	69.	B
6.	B	38.	C	70.	B
7.	B	39.	D	71.	C
8.	A	40.	C	72.	B
9.	D	41.	C	73.	C
10.	D	42.	D	74.	C
11.	D	43.	B	75.	D
12.	B	44.	B	76.	D
13.	C	45.	D	77.	A
14.	C	46.	D	78.	A
15.	B	47.	D	79.	B
16.	B	48.	A	80.	D
17.	C	49.	D	81.	C
18.	D	50.	A	82.	C
19.	B	51.	B	83.	A
20.	D	52.	D	84.	D
21.	B	53.	B	85.	D
22.	C	54.	B	86.	D
23.	C	55.	D	87.	A
24.	A	56.	B	88.	C
25.	D	57.	D	89.	B
26.	D	58.	A	90.	D
27.	D	59.	B	91.	B
28.	B	60.	D	92.	C
29.	A	61.	D	93.	B
30.	A	62.	D	94.	C
31.	C	63.	D	95.	B
32.	D	64.	C		

Chapter 14 Answers

1.	B		26.	D
2.	C		27.	C
3.	D		28.	D
4.	C		29.	C
5.	C		30.	C
6.	B		31.	C
7.	D		32.	C
8.	C		33.	C
9.	B		34.	C
10.	A		35.	A
11.	B		36.	B
12.	B		37.	D
13.	B		38.	C
14.	C		39.	D
15.	C		40.	A
16.	A		41.	C
17.	B		42.	A
18.	C		43.	B
19.	B		44.	A
20.	D		45.	A
21.	C		46.	D
22.	B		47.	A
23.	C		48.	C
24.	C		49.	A
25.	D		50.	A

Chapter 15 Answers

1.	D	36.	C
2.	B	37.	B
3.	A	38.	D
4.	D	39.	A
5.	B	40.	A
6.	D	41.	B
7.	B	42.	B
8.	C	43.	B
9.	A	44.	B
10.	D	45.	B
11.	B	46.	C
12.	A	47.	B
13.	C	48.	D
14.	D	49.	D
15.	A	50.	B
16.	D	51.	C
17.	C	52.	C
18.	B	53.	B
19.	A	54.	A
20.	D	55.	C
21.	D	56.	B
22.	D	57.	D
23.	C	58.	D
24.	D	59.	A
25.	B	60.	C
26.	C	61.	D
27.	C	62.	A
28.	B	63.	C
29.	B	64.	D
30.	A	65.	B
31.	A	66.	D
32.	C	67.	B
33.	D	68.	C
34.	A	69.	C
35.	C	70.	D

Chapter 16 Answers

1.	D	26.	B
2.	D	27.	D
3.	C	28.	A
4.	C	29.	D
5.	B	30.	C
6.	D	31.	C
7.	D	32.	C
8.	A	33.	C
9.	D	34.	B
10.	B	35.	D
11.	A	36.	C
12.	D	37.	A
13.	B	38.	C
14.	D	39.	D
15.	B	40.	B
16.	C	41.	D
17.	B	42.	B
18.	C	43.	D
19.	A	44.	C
20.	A	45.	C
21.	D	46.	C
22.	A	47.	D
23.	B	48.	D
24.	C	49.	D
25.	B	50.	C